TABLE OF CONTENTS

I0438762

INTRODUCTION

Eight years ago I did something I'd been wanting to do for a long time: I started meditating.

From my reading about meditation, I had the general idea that the goal of meditation is enlightenment. After eight years, I'm not enlightened, but I've learned a few things about meditation that I think are worth sharing.

One is that meditation is part of a way of life that is characterized by mindfulness. Mindfulness, like enlightenment, is a matter of degree, not like a light switch, Off or On. What I want to tell you about in this book is how a little mindfulness can go a long way when applied in a particular, targeted way. You don't have to be enlightened to begin to benefit from mindfulness. You don't even have to be an expert meditator.

In this book, I'm going to discuss a simple and relatively easy aspect of life: weight management. Some of the more basic and perhaps more difficult aspects are things like management of personal finances, or management of general health issues, or management of relationships.

Notice that I refer to weight management as "relatively easy." Some of us who have struggled for years to manage our weight might disagree with that description. What I mean is that in comparison to managing relationships, or general health, or for some people even money, managing our weight tends to engage fewer of our critical life issues. So if you are interested in personal change, it's easier to transform your body than it is to transform your relationships with all the people you know.

One point I want to insist on, though, is that mindfulness is an all-purpose tool for managing life's core issues. If you succeed, as I know you can, in following the simple guidance in this book, you won't just successfully manage your weight; you will have positioned yourself extremely well to follow that success with success in other areas of your life.

A meditation practice will support your practical attempts to manage any aspect of your life in a healthy direction. But it won't do it automatically. You can't expect to start meditating and just watch your life improve in all aspects. This book will give you simple step by step instructions both on how to start a meditation practice and how to apply your gradually acquired mindfulness to a specific area of your life: weight management.

This approach, by the way, is non-denominational. It's not based on accepting a particular religion or set of beliefs. Every religion I know of has some form of meditation practice, and no set of religious beliefs conflicts with the practice described and recommended here.

After a year or so of meditation, it occurred to me that I would be better off if I weighed ten pounds less. At that time I was tipping the scales at 186 or 187. I'm six feet tall, so that's not obese, but I thought 175 would be a healthier weight for me to carry for the rest of my life.

Since my forties I've been what's called a "yo-yo dieter." I would typically gain a pound or a pound and a half a month until I weighed more than I was comfortable with. Then I would cut back drastically on my food intake for a while, lose some weight, and then start the process over again. I refused to let myself get heavier than the low 190s, but was never able or adequately motivated to find a way to keep my weight where I wanted it, around 180.

As I began the process of getting down to 175, it became clear to me very soon that the process was qualitatively different from the other times I had lost weight. It didn't take long to discover that the difference was closely related to my meditation practice.

About four months after I decided to reduce my weight, I first saw 175 on my bathroom scale. This morning, over seven years later, I weighed 167.2, reflecting a subsequent decision to go down to 170.

Going from 186-187 to 175 was relatively easy, compared to the numerous times I lost weight before. Keeping the weight off hasn't been much of a problem either, and that's the main thing that's new. How I lost the 10-12 pounds, and later another five, and how I'm maintaining my weight at that level is what this book is about.

The only person I've talked to in any detail about the connection between mindfulness meditation and weight management is Art, my friend with whom I walk a 3 ½ mile route several times a week. During these walks any topic is fair game, and one night I mentioned that I weighed 180 pounds, and that I was on my way from 187 to 175.

Art was apparently intrigued by this, and kept bringing it up during subsequent walks. Why did I decide to lose weight? Why 175 pounds? What did I weigh this morning? How was I going about this weight loss? Art lives with my wife and me when he's in Hawaii, about six months out of the year, and he mentioned that he hadn't noticed any difference in my eating habits at the meals he shared with us.

Over time, under Art's probing, during the 180 to 175 part of my weight decline, I found myself articulating what turned out to be a surprisingly detailed but quite simple theory and practice of weight management. That's what gave me the impulse to write this book.

Neither weight management nor meditation is inherently very complicated, in spite of the many volumes devoted to both. In this book I'm going to take you way back to the basics of both. Even if you have had some experience with weight management, meditation, or both, if you are approaching this book with the serious intent to use my ideas and experience for your own benefit, you'll need to start at Step 1.

I'm going to assume, since you're reading this book, that if you were walking with Art and me you might have the same questions as Art, and I'm going to give you the full story. Maybe, like Art, you'll want at some point to borrow or buy a book or two I'll recommend about some elementary meditation practices. Maybe you'll buy a bathroom scale and take the simple steps I describe in Chapter One (Mindfulness First Steps) and Chapter Two (Weight Management First Steps).

Or maybe not. I don't think either Mindfulness or weight management is for everybody. If you think it might be for you and you take those all important first steps, I'd love to hear from you. How's it going? What's not as clear as it should be? What are you finding easy and what's difficult?

The best way to chat with me is on the blog I've set up for the readers of this book: mindfulnessmethodofweightmanagement.blogspot. com. If you have questions or want to share your experiences, the blog is a way to do those things and also potentially be helpful to other readers.

I. MINDFULNESS FIRST STEPS

Let me guess. You wanted me to start talking about weight management first. That's normal, especially in Western societies. We're results oriented. We want to cut to the chase, get to the bottom line. What do I need to do right now to manage my weight better?

My answer is: learn a little bit about meditation and mindfulness. That's the first step. Or if what you're really looking for is a diet book, the book stores are full of them. That's not what this book is.

There are lots of ways to get a start with meditation. My way may be too introverted for some of you. I'll describe my own approach in some detail, since that's what I know best, but will also try to give you some pointers for alternatives.

First the alternatives: all metropolitan areas have meditation centers of some sort. Most have quite a few, including several different approaches to meditation. The approach I'm most familiar with and most comfortable with is called Vipassana or Insight Meditation. There are also Transcendental Meditation and Zen and others. If you're interested in finding people who will teach you to meditate or who will meditate with you, do a little research on the web or the yellow pages and see what's available in your area.

If you're OK with starting out on your own, I recommend using one particular book as your guide: <u>Mindfulness in Plain English</u>, by Bhante

Henepola Gunaratana. There are many others, but this is the best introduction to meditation I've read. Another advantage is that the same author wrote a second book in the same user-friendly style that's a wonderful sequel: Eight Mindful Steps to Happiness. In Appendix A at the end of this book there's a short list of other books I've found useful over the past few years, and I'll tell you a little later how I use books as an aid to meditation.

These two books are excellent, and there are many others you can find that might suit you. For now I recommend against using the books about Zen meditation that are commonly found in American bookstores: Kapleau's The Three Pillars of Zen; and Zen: Merging of East and West; or Suzuki's Zen Mind, Beginner's Mind. Devotees of Zen may think I'm dead wrong about this, but for people with no previous experience and little personal knowledge of meditation, I think the Zen approach is a bit too hard core, and not as easy to get started without a teacher.

Until you get Mindfulness in Plain English and start to use it as a guide or manual, try getting started by taking the following steps:

- Sit comfortably in a place and at a time when you're not likely to be disturbed.
- Sit with your back straight. Everything else about how you sit is optional. You can use a chair or sit on a cushion on the floor with your legs crossed however you wish. If you sit on the floor, you'll find it important to your comfort to sit on something high and

firm enough that your butt is higher than your knees.

- Breathe.
- Pay attention to your breath.
- Breathe again. Follow your breath in and out, and pay attention only to your breath going in and out.
- Repeat the last step. Continue this for two or three minutes.

You have begun to meditate. You are being mindful of something: your breathing. You are not being mindful of anything else: what you need to do today; a conversation you had with your mother yesterday; where and what you plan to eat tonight.

What happened when you followed the directions above for a couple of minutes? Were you able to keep your full attention on your breath for more than a couple of breaths? If you were, congratulations. You're a fast learner.

If, as is usually the case, you found your mind losing track of your breath and wandering off to one of the hundreds of enticing topics it loves to dwell on, join the club. That's what the mind does. When that happens, all that's necessary is to notice it, and then return your focus, your mindfulness, to your breath.

When I did this exercise for the first time, a couple of things happened. One was that I was surprised at how hard it is to keep the mind focused on what's going on in the present, and how much the mind wants to be somewhere else. It wants to be in the past, or in the future, anywhere but the present moment, where I'm just sitting here watching my breath or experiencing something that's going on in my body or mind right now.

The second was an unexpected sense or feeling of relief, of relaxation, almost of nostalgia. It was as if turning my attention away from the automatic "thinking" the mind does when unattended was deeply restful, like coming home after a stressful day at the office.

Right now, after I wrote the last paragraph, I stopped and breathed mindfully for a couple of breaths, and there it was again: a kind of peacefulness, restfulness, homecoming. That's a natural, normal result of spending a few moments in the present. The breath is just a tool, a method of recalling my attention to the present, a way of helping myself be mindful of my present state of being.

A person could get hooked on this. And if that should happen to you, you would be a meditator. There are lots and lots of things going on in all our lives that work against this natural tendency, however, things that suck us back into our full time schedule of letting the "monkey mind" pull us here and there, from past to future and back to past, the mind run amok on automatic pilot.

That's why most if not all of us who are interested in discovering and returning to that quiet place where our motor-mouth brain is turned off for a little while need some special assistance to get there. That is, we need to develop habits that encourage and assist us in spending some time in that quiet, peaceful, restful place.

Here are a few things people have found useful:

- ✓ Set aside a time or times during the day when you always or usually do this. Some people like to do it in the morning before their regular day's activities begin. Some like to use a little time in the evening or night between dinner and bedtime. Or both.
- ✓ Use the same quiet place every day for your quiet time. Try to find a place that's easy, convenient, comfortable, and not likely to have heavy traffic from others.
- ✓ Don't start out trying to do this for very long. Five minutes or so is fine at the beginning. When you find that's not long enough, go ahead and extend it little by little, but don't do more than about twenty minutes at a time for the first several months.
- ✓ Don't be a meditation clock-watcher, but set a minimum time you want to stay in one position and be mindful of your breathing.
- ✓ Don't worry about what happens. There's nothing you're trying to achieve, no state of being you're trying to get to. Just pay attention and see what happens. And keep recalling your attention, your mindfulness, to your breathing process.

That's it for now. We'll get into more of the mechanics of mindfulness meditation as we go along, and we'll talk a little about the theory of meditation that's been developed over the centuries. But now we need to get to the first steps of weight management so we can develop mindfulness and weight management step by step together.

After you read the next chapter you'll be ready to start the first two weeks of your introduction to the mindfulness method of weight management. Meanwhile, make sure to find at least a few minutes each day to practice mindfulness of breathing.

If you're not too eager to charge ahead, you might wait a week before you read the next chapter. That would give you time to begin to form the habit of meditation, maybe just five minutes once or twice a day at first. In any case, whether you go on to the next chapter immediately or not, it's critical that you begin now to spend some bit of time, however small, following the meditation instructions above each day.

Mindful Message: When you meditate, you are storing up a special kind of personal energy, which you can apply to any area of your life you choose.

II. WEIGHT MANAGEMENT FIRST STEPS

It's impossible to miss the fact that an awful lot of people these days have problems with weight management. Not just because weight problems tend to be very visible, but also because in general conversations weight comes up so often. Individually and as a society we've become obsessed with the topic.

Bill Clinton's hamburger habit, George Bush's workout regimen, Barack Obama's leanness, the issue of childhood obesity, a jillion books about diets, Diet Fad One through One Hundred: the issue of weight **as a problem** is front and center in this country and much of the rest of the "developed" world.

Since I started writing this book I've become more aware of all the attention weight loss gets. There are probably a million ads on the Internet promoting some method of weight loss. When I'm checking out in the grocery store line, I can usually spot ten or twelve magazine covers that use the promise of special diets to sell themselves.

This book will not present any complicated theories of diet or weight management. It will reduce weight management to its simplest components, just as Chapter I began by reducing the first principles of mindfulness to simple steps related to the simple act of breathing and directing the mind's attention to breathing.

Both mindfulness and weight management are very simple at their cores. This idea may seem to be contradicted by the large number of complicated theories spelled out in great detail in shelves full of books. However, for now please assume that you don't need to know very much about either meditation or diet. Just take these simple steps with me and pay attention to what happens.

If you don't already have one, purchase a bathroom scale. It should be digital, and it should show your weight to the tenth of a pound.

If you don't already maintain a planning calendar for your work or personal use, you'll need to get some kind of calendar so you can record your weight every day.

This chapter tells you how to operate your weight management program for the first two weeks. That means that: (1) you need to have made a decision that you are going to start a weight management program based on this book; and (2) that you have a scale and a calendar and have decided that some specific date is the first day of the two week period.

Part of the power of mindfulness is intentionality. That's why as we begin to talk about weight management, I'll insist that you act with deliberateness and attention. The more explicit you are with yourself about your intention, the better your focus and attention will be. So don't drift along from step to step. Tell yourself clearly, if that's your intention, that you are going to start your program next week Monday, or the first of next month.

If your intention is just to read through this book first before deciding to do anything, make that intention explicit to yourself. Then when you are ready to start the program, come back here and explicitly make the intention to start.

For the first two weeks, it's important not to try to lose any weight. You're just going to use these two weeks to learn to pay attention to certain aspects of weight as they apply to you.

On Day One, when you get up in the morning, do your normal waking up routine. Brush your teeth, pee, take a shower, whatever you normally do, and then weigh yourself. You should be naked when you do this, unless you want to fool your scale tomorrow by wearing lighter pajamas. Then weigh yourself again. If you get a different weight the second time, weigh yourself again until you get the same reading twice in a row.

Scales can be affected by all sorts of things: temperature; position on the floor; balance; being bumped, etc. Weighing yourself in this precise way gives your scale a chance to work out its issues and give you a reasonably accurate number.

Write down the result on your calendar.

Notice your reaction to your weight. Try to just "barely notice" your reaction; don't dwell on it. Are you happy? Satisfied? Horrified? Disgusted? Try to notice and maybe give a name to your reaction. What's important is to pay attention not only or even mainly to the particular number you just saw on your scale, but to your reaction or feeling about the number. Then try to let it go. It's just information you're after here: information about your weight, and information about your attitude to it.

You'll be doing this same drill each morning of the first two weeks. You're not trying to make the numbers come out one way or the other; you're not even concerned whether the number you see today is higher or lower than the one you saw yesterday.

Now while you're following the directions in this chapter during this two week period, you're also practicing the mindfulness techniques described in the last chapter. Each day you're spending some time, no less than five minutes, paying attention to your breathing while you're sitting with your back straight. And you're doing something about getting your hands on <u>Mindfulness in Plain English</u> or some other introduction to Insight Meditation.

There's only one more thing you need to do during this first two weeks.

Pay attention to your eating patterns. Try to do this with as little judgment as possible.

Do you generally have the same breakfast each morning? Do you always have breakfast at all? In this first two weeks, what variations in your breakfasting do you notice? Did you have fourteen different breakfasts? Three? Do you rotate them? How do you decide what to have for breakfast? Do you generally eat breakfast out or at home?

We tend to take our own routines for granted. So I'm just asking you to pay gentle, non-critical attention to your food routines.

If you're a little on the obsessive side and you want to write down what you observe, it's OK to do that. I don't recommend getting into a full scale food diary at this point. You may never need to.

Pay the same kind of attention to lunch and dinner. And pay attention to what happens between breakfast, lunch, and dinner. Is your food intake pretty much limited to those three occasions each day, or is there some snacking between the organized meal times? What kinds of snacks do you keep stocked in your home or office? What's your favorite snack? How often do you snack?

Again, don't try to change anything. Just pay attention to what is.

For now, meaning the first two weeks of your new program, just religiously follow the instructions above. When you're done with that, check back in with me for new directions in the next two chapters. **It's best if you don't read ahead.**

If at the end of the two week period you find that you only found a few minutes to meditate four or five times out of the fourteen days, or you only remembered to weigh and record your weight five or six times, don't go ahead with Chapters III and IV.

I can't emphasize too much the importance of precisely following the directions for the first two weeks before you go ahead. If you didn't succeed in your first attempt, simply notice that, pay attention to whatever kept you from succeeding, and then go back, set a new beginning day for your next two-week attempt, and try it again.

What you're being asked to do during the first two weeks of this program may seem too simple and easy for you to take seriously. You might be tempted to skip forward and go ahead with the next steps. If so, resist the temptation. What you are being asked to do is of huge importance. I even encourage you to re-read this chapter and Chapter I over again between Week I and Week II to make sure you're covering everything.

People like to say: "I'm just not disciplined enough to do X," as if being disciplined were some internal quality some people are lucky enough to have and others don't. I've heard people say: "I could never meditate; my mind is way too active," as if only they are burdened with the chattering monkey mind.

We're not talking about internal qualities here.

People who claim to lack discipline can be observed to have certain routines or habits that they honor regardless of whatever else is going on. I know people who claim to lack discipline who never miss a particular TV show or recreational activity that they value. Their discipline with regard to their own habits and preferences is awesome.

The power of habits, sometimes called "habit energy," is tremendous. You have it. You have excellent discipline. It may or may not be at your service in exactly the way you wish.

So don't think of the few simple things I have so far asked you to do as requiring any special qualities that you don't have. **Just do the actions! The discipline will take care of itself.** If you choose not to do one or another of the things I'm asking you to do, just say to yourself: "I choose not to do that," and acknowledge to yourself that if you don't follow the recipe, you can't expect the cake.

Mindful Message: Just do the actions. The discipline will take care of itself. In two weeks, you'll be fully equipped for what comes next.

III. SOME MINDFULNESS BASICS

In this chapter I want to cover some basic practical matters related to the physical practice of meditation. Then I'll give you a Meditation 101 summary of a couple of theoretical matters.

I'm trying to thread my way between two extremes here. I don't want to make this a full course in meditation; that's why I've encouraged you to choose another book to flesh out the skeleton I'm giving you. But I do want to give you enough basic information about meditation and mindfulness to tie in with the specific recommendations I'm making in this book about weight management.

First, some mechanical stuff.

Meditation is not about endurance, nor is it about learning to tolerate pain or even discomfort for extended periods of time. However, sitting still for more than 15 seconds can be challenging for some of us, and sitting with our backs straight can go against a whole lifetime of dedicated slouching.

Both sitting still and sitting with our backs straight work much better with some good basic equipment. Most meditators sit on the floor rather than on a chair, and to sit on the floor comfortably you need two things: some kind of mat or cushion to keep your ankle bones from grinding against a hard floor; and a cushion to sit on so that your butt is higher than your knees. If the place you've chosen to meditate has a thick carpet or the equivalent, you may be able to skip the pad.

There is a firm round cushion designed for meditation called a zafu. If you're in a large city, you probably can find a shop that carries meditation supplies, including zafus. If not, there are numerous websites where you can order them. I recently bought both a meditation cushion and a zafu from dharmacrafts.com for about $100. Their website also has a page called "meditation instruction" which has some helpful descriptions and pictures of correct sitting posture.

Once you get these things, experiment with various cross-legged positions until you find one that's reasonably comfortable. If you want to, you can work up to a specialized mediation position like the half lotus or full lotus position later. Like much of the meditation paraphernalia you'll see in shops and on web pages, these specialized positions are not essential for getting started.

Now for two bits of basic meditation theory.

As you begin a meditation practice, you'll find as thousands of meditation beginners have found before you that your focus will move back and forth between two essential elements of meditation: concentration (sometimes referred to as calm or focus) on the one hand, and awareness or insight on the other.

Because these modes of experience, and the movement between them, lie outside the common conscious experience of most people, I want to lay out in some detail what to expect, and why this is so important for the benefits you can expect to realize from meditation.

Insight arises out of the calm of concentration. It's not a matter of figuring out anything, or "thinking through" anything. Rather, insights into your life and your patterns of living, thinking, feeling, and acting will arise of themselves, a by-product of concentration, focus, and calm.

Concentration itself, as experienced in meditation, is almost the opposite of what we usually think of as concentration. It's not a matter of focusing your mind like a laser on something. Concentration or calm is primarily the practice and the result of shutting down or diminishing the constant flow of chatter in the monkey mind.

Have you ever had the experience of being in a large space full of people, all of them talking away in groups and couples, and then something happens that causes everybody to stop talking at the same time? The contrast between the sound of everybody talking and the "sound" of everybody being silent is similar to the difference between your mind carrying on the normal subliminal commentary that constitutes the ego's normal pursuits and the "self" in a state of calm concentration.

When you start meditating, you may find yourself constantly becoming aware that you have lost mindfulness of your breath, and that you have somehow gotten inside a mental conversation about something or other that happened in the past or that you anticipate happening in the future.

The practice of concentration in meditation involves the constant recall of your attention or mindfulness to your breathing or to some other present object of mindfulness. This mental wandering and recall can happen dozens of times in even a short meditation session. It's completely normal.

Each time it happens, there's actually a double activity. The first is that you become mindful that your monkey mind is at it again, and you can notice, without getting hung up on it, what it is that the monkey mind has found to play with. The second is that you choose to pull your attention away from whatever it is and again focus on your breathing.

As this happens, you will notice that the patterns or topics the monkey mind lapses back into can be pretty easily categorized. The categories you begin to get familiar with as a result of this awareness form a list of your favorite pre-occupations. For example, here are a couple of categories of mental games my monkey mind loves to get into: (1) the details of what I'm going to do with my day; (2) imaginary conversations with people with whom I have issues, in which I instruct and advise them as to the proper way to deal with their lives; (3) various scenarios related to playing and teaching Bridge; (4) arguments or justifications with people against whom I am currently harboring various resentments or anger.

I assume that each meditator after a few months of meditating can construct his or her own list of favorite monkey mind activities. Becoming more aware of these habitual patterns of ego activity is itself a valuable form of insight.

Now why is such a simple and repetitious mental exercise of any importance? What is it supposed to achieve?

To answer that question, we first have to understand something about the monkey mind: specifically, what it does, and why it does it. The second thing we have to get clear on is how and why the monkey mind **is not us**, which we'll get into later in this chapter.

What I am calling the monkey mind is a hugely important aspect of the normal human brain. It is a part of the brain that talks to itself with the primary purpose of creating your individual reality or world and maintaining it. Some people refer to this function as "self talk." Some people call a part of it the Super Ego; that's the part that you'll catch lecturing you and trying to enforce some basic moral premises that you may or may not consciously subscribe to.

You can have varying degrees of awareness of this function. Certainly you are not aware of it all the time. That is, it continues to do what it does whether "you" are consciously aware of it or not. That's why you may be surprised sometime when you suddenly become aware that there's a whole conversation going on in your mind that you only become conscious of somewhere in the middle of the conversation. If you start paying more attention to this function, you'll catch your monkey mind in the middle of a sentence, the beginning of which you may or may not be able to remember. You may recognize echoes of a parent's voice, or the phrasing of an author you've been reading.

Think of the mental space where the monkey mind resides as "the spin room." This function is constantly commenting on everything in your world, interpreting what's going on, making sure that whatever you experience forms the consistent tissue that you have come to understand as your universe. It explains to you why you are right and other people are wrong. It justifies the fact that your actions, while perhaps appearing to be unacceptable, were actually unavoidable, or were necessary because of something somebody else did. It's the place where all the psychological defenses we have—denial, projection, displacement—have their home.

It's also the place where the part of you that feels guilty scolds the part of you that has transgressed. It's the place where you voice your worries, and the worrying voice can continue even while you're doing something else with your conscious mind, or while you're sleeping.

However important this function is to our consciousness, one of the insights meditation can lead to is the clear realization that the monkey mind is not me. It's not the only, or highest, or most central aspect of what I call my self.

Getting some practical separation from the persistent, insistent, demanding, neurotic, egoistic, fearful, petulant, rationalizing, judgmental, opinionated voice of the monkey mind is one of the primary valuable results of meditation.

Here's the crux of this matter. What we normally think of as insight and even as mindfulness actually falls within the purview of the monkey mind. When we "realize" something, or "come to an understanding" of something, what is actually happening is that we're partially controlling this ego-function with the result that its contents are slightly rearranged. We substitute one opinion for another. We come to a new understanding or realization on some topic.

If you have read this book from cover to cover and understand it completely, you have not yet taken Step I of the process of mindfulness or meditation that I am advocating. **You can only take Step I when you initiate the practice of regular meditation.** That's when you begin to develop the kind of mindfulness and insight that I believe is critically important for any type of serious personal change or improvement, whether it be successful management of weight, or management of money, or management of relationships.

Mindfulness is not thinking about what you're doing. It's not just directing your attention to your eating, your spending, or your conversations with your spouse or lover. That kind of "paying attention" is largely conducted by the ego or monkey mind.

The insight you're after in meditation is only partly intellectual; that's the least important part of it. **The most important insights occur somewhere in your being other than in your manipulative mind, and those insights become meaningful to you as subtle but powerful shifts in your way of seeing and living.** Insight as a result of meditation is just as physical as it is mental, and it is just as spiritual as it is physical. **It is facilitated by stopping the ego talk, by interrupting the monkey mind, even for one second.**

Remember that the ego talk has been going on for almost as many years as you have been alive, and it has important functions in your life. It's not going to stop just because you want it to. However, you can, through the practice of meditation, begin to interrupt it for brief periods of time, sometimes only seconds at a time. That's the beginning of real change. It's a way of creating or saving a special type of psychic or psychological or personal energy which generates deep physical, intellectual and spiritual insights that slowly and gradually allow you to change your life.

Getting your arms around those concepts may take a little time; it may even require a significant amount of time meditating and trying to live a mindful life. Human beings are pretty complicated, so there's no point pretending that understanding what happens with mindfulness is simple and easy to grasp. Plan to come back to this chapter and reread it as you get deeper into your meditation practice.

Another way to think about the process of meditation is to start with the question: Who am I? Am I a composite of a body and a soul? A body and a mind? Pay attention to whatever you consider the components of your "self."

Are you the mind that you've noticed keeps up a constant chatter to itself whether "you" are paying attention or not? In this book we've been referring to that function of the brain or mind as the "monkey mind" or the ego.

Are you the entity or being that is capable of being aware of both your body and your monkey mind? The being that is capable of being mindful? Can you notice that there's even a level of "you" that's capable of being aware of the "you" that's being mindful of the monkey mind?

Are you in control of your body? In what sense is it "your" body if you're not in control of it? How about your mind?

Are you a composite of your thoughts and emotions?

One way of looking at insight meditation is that it's a very detailed, almost clinical, way of examining in a mostly non-conceptual way your relationship to all the aspects of what we normally think of as "me" and "mine."

That's one piece of theory about meditation or mindfulness. It's not something that's useful to obsess about. It is a foundational aspect of insight meditation that I want you to be familiar with. Learning to be mindful of the "monkey mind" as a constant presence that is not you and that can be observed and managed as something separate from a larger you is a critical and eminently practical lesson. Here's a second.

The basic model of meditation that starts with observing the breath is a formally structured framework that's been worked out over several thousand years. That model has four sets of four steps, a total of sixteen steps. <u>Mindfulness in Plain English</u> is a modern exposition of those sixteen steps.

Here I'm going to give you a super-brief description of that system so you'll know the focus on the breath is not a stand-alone gimmick.

The first set of four steps focuses on the body and the ways the breath affects the body, and the ways changes in the body affect the breathing process.

The second set of four steps relates to feelings, which are affected by the breath and the body. These steps get into very detailed work with the emotions.

The third set of four steps relates to the mind, which is affected by the emotions, which are affected by the body, which is affected by the breath.

You start to get the picture. We start with the breath because it's a convenient place to start, but we work our way up through the natural dynamics of human nature from lower and simpler to higher and more complex functions.

The fourth set of four steps involves aspects of the nature of reality. By the time we get to this final set of four, the theory goes, we will have tools— body, emotions, and mind—that are capable of and trained for the perception of reality or truth.

In practice, it's not so clear cut and linear. But even as you start playing with the first steps, involving mindfulness of the breath, it can be helpful to understand the overall structure of the meditation process.

Hopefully by now you've gotten <u>Mindfulness in Plain English</u> and have started reading it. Maybe you've set aside some bit of time each day to focus on being mindful of your breathing. You might even have gotten a cushion and zafu and have organized a place for your meditation.

At the least, if you are approaching mindfulness with some degree of seriousness, you have been spending at least a few minutes a day doing absolutely nothing but paying attention to your breathing.

That's good for now. I want to make just one more suggestion before going on to cover some weight management basics so that your mindfulness practice and your application of mindfulness to weight management keep a healthy pace with each other.

That suggestion is to keep in mind that reading about meditation is totally secondary to actually meditating. Some of us are concept hogs. Put a book in our hands and we just want to plow through it, understand it, and put it aside. We gulp it down without truly experiencing it, just as we may do our food. Just the opposite is called for here.

Some religious disciplines refer to "spiritual reading." That's what we're aiming at here. Read the book you've chosen very slowly, as if in slow motion. Use it to put yourself in a mental and emotional state suitable for meditation.

My own morning ritual goes like this. I do some simple floor stretches and exercises to get the blood flowing and to make sure my muscles and joints are still functional. Then while I have my first cup of tea, I read whatever book about meditation I'm reading at the time. I read only as long as it takes to finish the cup of tea. Then I head for my screened gazebo for meditation.

Used in this way, the book is a kind of transition from being semi-asleep to being in a condition suitable for meditation.

Work out your own way to use the book to support the meditation. The critical thing is to remember that meditation is the thing. Understanding some concepts about meditation is more or less worthless unless it's a lead-in to practice.

Mindful Message: Learning to be mindful of the "monkey mind" as a constant presence that is not you and that can be observed and managed as something separate from a larger you is a critical and eminently practical lesson.

IV. SOME WEIGHT MANAGEMENT BASICS

I want to start this chapter by mentioning a couple of things you no doubt already know, but that are important to have front and center in your attention as we go on to the next steps. These next few paragraphs, by the way, are about as technical as I'm going to get.

A calorie is a unit of energy. When food is oxidized or "burned" in the body, it produces energy. A calorie is a measure of the amount of energy a certain amount of food produces when burned in the body. A calorie is also taken to mean the amount of food it takes to produce that specific amount of energy.

There's an equivalence between calories and weight. Specifically, the amount of food you need to consume in order to gain one pound is about 3600 calories.

If I consume each day exactly the amount of food that it takes to generate the amount of energy I use up that day, I will neither gain nor lose any pounds. This is true regardless of body type, metabolism, level of activity, or type of food eaten.

What causes me to gain weight is consuming more calories than I burn.

What causes me to lose weight is burning more calories than I consume.

Obviously, if I want to lose weight, I have two main choices: I can consume fewer calories or I can burn more calories.

For reasons I'll get into later, I'm asking you to forget about option 2 most of the time. Burning more calories is a fine thing, but as a primary strategy for managing weight, it's a sure road to frustration, for reasons I'll explain.

Now let's pick up where we left off at the end of Chapter II.

You've got your tools, and you've weighed yourself every day for two weeks, and you've recorded your weight each day. In addition, you've become a regular meditator, spending at least five minutes at a time, once or twice a day, focusing your attention specifically and exclusively on your breath. You may have missed a day or two during the past two weeks, either in weighing yourself and recording your weight or in your meditation practice, but overall this paragraph describes where you are.

If the previous paragraph is not an accurate description, I strongly recommend that you go back to the previous chapters, begin your two week pre-beginning period again, and make sure that you meet the description in the last paragraph before you read further.

Now the preparation is over, and it's time to start your active program. This is best done on a Monday, and from now on we will refer to a week as running from Monday morning when you get up to Sunday night when you go to bed.

This Monday morning your weight was whatever your scale told you it was. That's probably within a pound or two of the average of the weights you recorded during the two week preparation period. But we'll think and talk about this weight as your beginning weight.

By itself, it's not a very meaningful number, but I'm pretty sure that it has significance for you. And that's as it should be. Your weight is the precise and inevitable result of quite a large number of important factors in your life.

Why do you weigh exactly what you weigh on Day 1? I'd like you to spend some time thinking about that over the next few days. Are there some specific physical causes that affect your weight? Some genetic factors, perhaps? Sometimes body types run in families. Some metabolic factors? Sometimes people say "It's really hard for me to control my weight because my metabolism is slow." That usually means "Because of the way my body burns calories, it takes more exercise or work for me to burn the same number of calories as most other people."

Are there any psychological reasons for your weight to be what it is? What kind of psychological factors do you think affect weight, and your own weight in particular? Some people say they eat more when they're tense or nervous, and eating calms them down. Some people say they suffer from guilt feelings, and eating helps keep the guilt under control. Some people say they eat more when they're angry.

My point in having you focus on this issue is that everybody's weight is what it is for a host of reasons that are sufficient and necessary to produce in them precisely whatever they weigh. **You weigh what you weigh for excellent reasons. Those reasons are different for each of us**. The mindfulness method of weight management doesn't require you to analyze or understand all of them, but don't be surprised if you discover quite a bit about the causes and effects of your weight before you get through this process.

What is important is that you realize your weight is not an accident. It's pure cause and effect, even though some of the causes can be quite complex.

If you weigh precisely what you weigh this first Monday morning for excellent reasons, what do you think might happen if you reduce your weight by, say, ten pounds. If some of the reasons you used to weigh ten pounds more were physical, you might start feeling some physical repercussions of that weight loss. If some of the reasons were psychological, you might start feeling some emotional or psychological or psychosomatic repercussions of losing ten pounds. Sometimes the mere **intention** to do something about your weight can trigger reactions that feel like your body or your "self" retaliating against your own intention.

What's almost certain is that your own personal set of physical and psychological factors that caused you to weigh what you weighed on Day 1 will at some point manifest itself. These factors or causes will pull you and push you in a hundred subtle ways to get back to the weight you started at, because based on those physical and psychological factors, that was the "right" weight for you. You may have already experienced this if you've made previous attempts to lose weight and keep it off.

This is a dynamic that is at work in that common pattern of dieting and losing weight, and then gaining the weight back, commonly called "yo-yo dieting." Your self-control, exercised through your conscious mind and your will power, allow you to control your diet enough to lose some weight. Then your whole physical and psychological and spiritual self gradually reasserts itself in the physical form of your "right" weight.

To counteract that set of factors, you can do one or both of two things. You can continue to resist those factors through further exercise of "will power" or "mind control" or "discipline." **Or/and you can change some of the physical and psychological factors that affect your weight.** The mindfulness method of weight management is designed to coach you and to help you coach yourself to do both. Using this method, you will most likely lose some weight and then at some point you'll deal with the factors that control weight in such a way as to de-activate or weaken or change some of the factors that have in the past caused you to gain weight back.

Now let's go back to Day 1. You weigh X pounds, and you have recorded that weight on your calendar.

Let's assume the number you recorded is higher than you would like it to be. In fact, to make the process easier to talk about, let's say the number was 162. That sounds like a pretty good weight, except that based on the height of the person we're going to make up and use as an example (Example Person) and based on her doctor's advice, her ideal weight would be 132. To make it worse, Example Person(EP) has considered herself significantly overweight for years, and has tried six different diets. In spite of her best efforts, she has gained 5 pounds over the past year, and 10 pounds over the past two years. She's had a couple of six-month periods where her weight stabilized or she even lost a few pounds, but those pounds came back with interest.

Whenever I talk about EP, it's just because it's easier to make my points using specifics. You can always substitute your own data, and I advise you to do so.

Whatever the details of your situation, I think it's ill advised to worry about "ideal weight" or even long term goals at this point. Let's set those matters aside and plan to worry about them later. Instead, for now, let's think only about the next one month period.

Think about what it means to lose a pound. It means that over some period of time, you need to consume 3600 fewer calories than you need to maintain your current weight. If you're currently gaining weight, it also means that you first need to stop consuming more calories than you need to maintain your weight, and on top of that you need to reduce your calorie intake by 3600 additional calories. Whenever you do that, however long it takes, you will for sure lose one pound.

If it takes 2000 calories per day to maintain your weight, and you are currently consuming 2100 calories per day, you will gain a new pound every 36 days. If instead you want to lose a pound in the next 36 days, you must not only stop consuming the extra 100 calories per day, you have to cut an additional 100 calories per day, down to 1900 calories per day. If you do that, you will inevitably lose a pound over the next 36 days.

Remember that what we're doing right now is thinking about setting a goal for only the next one month. That first goal should be modest, but not too modest. If it's too modest, success will not be exciting, and it's important for success to be exciting. It's the mind we're after here. If we're successful in getting the mind to line up with our goals, the body will follow along. And the mind feeds on satisfaction. If you're achieving a goal that doesn't satisfy the mind, the achievement won't last.

The important thing is to find out what the right pace is for you. This first one month period is where you experiment with that. So hypothetically, let's set a goal that would be exciting to achieve but appears modest enough to be achievable. Would you be excited if, at the end of a month, you had lost a pound that you could count on not gaining back?

Now this may not sound very exciting. After all, I could find a dozen diets that promise to have you drop ten or fifteen pounds in a month or less. But if you are at all typical of the many, many people who have been concerned about their weight for a long time, you've already tried those diets and have either failed to lose the promised weight, or have lost it and gained it back.

The truth is, for a number of excellent reasons the slow, patient approach to weight management is the surest and healthiest approach. Speed is the enemy. Many "experts" on weight management suggest a much more radical approach that what I am recommending. If your goal is to get your weight to the level you consider appropriate for you, and then to keep it there, I strongly recommend that you at least start out thinking in terms of one pound per month. If you succeed, as I am confident you can, in maintaining that rate of loss for three months, that will be the time to re-evaluate your goals. In three months, you will have significantly more experience and knowledge of the mindfulness method of weight management.

Think about it this way. When was the last time you weighed twelve pounds less than you weighed on Day 1 of this program? If, one year from today, you could weigh twelve pounds less than you do now, and in addition you could count on continuing to permanently lose another pound each month until you were satisfied with your weight, would that prospect excite you?

In the case of EP, if she could lose a pound a month, it would be an impressive accomplishment, and it would bode well for her future additional goals. If she could lose twelve pounds over twelve months, she could expect to be at her doctor's recommended weight of 132 in two years and a half.

If you work out the arithmetic, you'll see that losing a pound a month means reducing your calorie intake by about 120 calories per day below what it would take to maintain your current weight. That seems like quite a bit. If you have been gaining weight over the past several years, you know that you must be presently consuming more calories per day than it takes to maintain your weight at the same level. If you've been doing that at the level of only 50 calories per day (one pound gained every 2 ½ months), you're now looking at cutting your caloric intake by 120 calories per day plus 50 calories per day. That's 8½ percent below what you would need to eat to maintain your weight at the same level.

Notice the balancing you're doing in your mind as you go about setting your goal and your intention for the first month. If you're EP, you know that if you continue as you've been doing for the past two years, at the end of the next three months you'll weigh not 162 but 163.5 pounds. So maybe it's exciting enough to set the goal of being at 161 pounds at the end of the first month, 160 at the end of two months, and 159 at the end of three months. By that time she'll have more experience and more practice of mindfulness, and perhaps can set a more ambitious goal for the following months.

Remember that if you succeed in reaching your one-month goal, you will have accomplished something ten times more important than the number of pounds you will have lost or not gained.

You will have begun to answer a critical question: Who is in charge here? Who determines what I will weigh? Who makes the decisions that determine what I will weigh?

Is it the food marketing industry? Is it the person who prepares the snacks? Is it the co-worker who brings in the donuts? Is it my Monkey Mind? Hell no! I'm in charge. I make the decisions. (And who is the "I" here if it's not your Monkey Mind? That's the mystery question we'll look at later.)

That's enough for right now. You've made the decision and set the intention of using the mindfulness method to lose some weight; you've done some careful thinking about the mechanics of weight loss in terms of calories; you've established some baseline information about your weight without excessive judgment; you've reached Day 1 of your program; and you've set a goal for the first month.

You have also developed some interesting information about your current eating habits, some of it probably new to you, some of it perhaps surprising.

In addition, you've taken the first steps toward creating a meditation or mindfulness practice in your life.

That's a lot. You haven't yet lost any weight, but you've laid a good foundation for what comes next. In my opinion, nothing you'll be called on to do in the next three months is any harder than what you've already accomplished.

If you haven't noticed, I want to point out that here we are at the end of Chapter IV, and you have not yet been asked to do anything at all different than what you've done in the past as far as your eating is concerned. Everything you've been asked to do has been in your head. There's an important message in that. **The most important things you have needed to do up to this point, and the most important things you will need to do in the future are all in your head.**

How well positioned you will be when you get to Chapter VI, where you will be asked to start doing some physical things different than you do them now, depends on what you are doing with your mind now. The more seriously you are practicing your meditation, the more mindfulness and personal energy you will have at your disposal as you start actually changing behaviors and habits.

Mindful Message: If you succeed in reaching your one-month goal, even if it seems quite modest to you, you will have accomplished something ten times more important than the number of pounds you have lost or not gained. You will have begun to answer a critical question: Who is in charge here?

Chapter V. Mindfulness and the Mouth

In this chapter we will begin to make the linkage between mindfulness and weight management more explicit.

The philosophy and psychology underlying Vipassana meditation is that of the Buddhist tradition. This has little to do with "religion" in the Western sense.

The Buddha is reported to have characterized his entire teaching as being about suffering and the end of suffering. The human condition, according to Buddhism, is characterized by suffering, but suffering is conditional, not necessary. There are natural causes of suffering. A correct understanding of how the world works and skillful actions in keeping with that understanding can reduce or even eliminate suffering.

Understanding the operations of cause and effect as they apply to suffering and happiness means understanding the Path that leads from suffering to happiness. This Path or Way is called The Eightfold Path. This Path is described in detail in one of the books listed at the end of this book: Eight Mindful Steps to Happiness, by Bhante Henepola Gunaratana.

The eight steps are: Skillful Understanding; Skillful Thinking; Skillful Speech; Skillful Action; Skillful Livelihood; Skillful Effort; Skillful Mindfulness; and Skillful Concentration.

"Skillful" just means "effective." These steps are considered necessary and sufficient to lead a person from suffering to happiness.

The Bible means the same thing when it says "As you sow, so shall you reap." Perhaps the main difference in the Buddhist approach is that there's little emphasis on moral judgment, and more emphasis on cause and effect.

In this chapter I want to suggest two ways for you to begin to experiment with this concept. The first has to do specifically with your meditation practice. The second has to do with eating. Both are about mindfulness, and both have something to do with moving from suffering to happiness.

First, let's review.

At this point, you have begun a more or less formal and systematic practice of meditation. At a minimum, you are spending a short period of time every day or almost every day focusing solely on your breathing. When you are distracted by thoughts or awareness of feelings, you are gently returning your mindfulness to your breath.

Perhaps in addition you have gotten the book I recommended, and have started using it as a primer for your practice. Maybe you have gotten a zafu and found a regular place and time for meditation.

If you have not taken action to accomplish what I describe above as the minimum, I recommend that you take stock of your intentions. Have you concluded that this approach is not for you? Do you think fulfilling the minimum requirements is too burdensome to be worth giving a try? Do you think of yourself as just checking out the concepts of this book in an abstract way before you start actually doing anything?

The approach to weight management presented in this book is not primarily conceptual. It's experiential and experimental. It's based on taking certain simple actions and paying attention to what happens as a result. It's about cause and effect. If you are serious about the mindfulness method of weight management and you haven't been able to give the method five to ten minutes a day of mindfulness practice, you may well have already discovered a lack of intention that will be fatal to any attempt to manage your physical condition. I recommend that you go back and start over with the first chapter, or that you explicitly conclude that you're not really ready to do anything about the issues that brought you to this book.

Clarity with yourself about your intentions is essential.

If you have met at least the minimum participation requirements, you're well-positioned to move forward with the second tier of critical steps. Here we go.

First step. In the time you devote to meditation, begin to pay some attention not only to the process of breathing, but to your body. Pay attention to the connection between the way you are breathing and how your body feels.

Have you ever been told: "Take a deep breath." Or "Remember to breath." These are expressions of a folk wisdom acknowledging the connection between mindful breathing and physical, emotional, and mental well-being.

Is there a difference in how you feel overall when your breathing is smooth, slow, and fine, and when it is rough, fast, and coarse? As you relax and let go of concerns and worries and plans, do you notice your breath getting longer and finer? If you notice that you are nervous or agitated, whether in your meditation or throughout the day, try slowing down your breathing and taking deeper, longer breaths for a minute. See what happens.

Also, as you are sitting, let your attention scan your body and see how it's doing. Are you comfortable? Does something hurt? Are you settled into your posture, or do you feel like fidgeting? Let your attention dwell for a minute on any part of your body that's clamoring for attention. Is there a tense shoulder or neck? An aching back? A knee that's not yet accustomed to the cross-legged position?

Just notice this area briefly without letting your mind get into making up a story about it. This is a technique called "barely noticing" something. It's just a sensory, non-conceptual, non-judgmental noticing. Then shift your mindfulness back to your breath. There's a Buddhist saying: Pain is inevitable; suffering is optional. Noticing mild pain or discomfort without getting into a big mental concern or worry about it is a way to experience the difference.

For all its incredible speed and flexibility, you'll find that the mind can only be attentive to one thing at a time. It can switch from one thing to another with such rapidity that it can seem to be multi-tasking, but it's really just being mindful of one thing at a time.

Notice what happens to the perception of pain or discomfort when you move your mindfulness back to the breath.

What you're doing is playing with cause and effect as they relate to breathing and other physical and mental functions. You can do this during your meditation sessions and from time to time throughout the day.

That's it for now. Now for the part about food and mindfulness.

Different cultures have different attitudes toward food. Think about the difference between British and French cuisine. Historically as well as geographically there are huge differences in attitudes toward food.

Is food for you primarily about nourishment? About survival? About entertainment? Is food just fuel for the physical machine, or is it nourishment for the soul?

Here's a simple experiment I'd like you to perform. Don't worry; this isn't a test you can fail.

Take a grape or some other piece of food that you can manage in one bite. Hold it in your hand and feel its texture. Notice how it feels in your fingers when you squeeze it a little.

Take a close look at it. Is it the same color all over? Are there any blemishes? How does the part look where it was attached to the vine?

Form the intention of putting it in your mouth. Notice how your arm and hand respond, and how your arm/hand movements are coordinated with getting your mouth ready to receive it.

Move the grape around in your mouth for a minute without biting into it. Does it have a taste before the skin in broken? Notice how perceptive your tongue is to the texture.

Bite into it once, and then hold it there. What happens? Can you feel your salivary ducts do their thing? What's going on with taste? With perception of texture?

Chew it up very slowly. Notice how you automatically move it to the part of your mouth that's most efficient at smashing and grinding. Notice how juicy it is. How the juice from the fruit and the saliva stimulated by the taste combine. (As I write this, I'm noticing how I'm getting the salivary part, even without the grape.)

Swallow the grape. Notice the taste remaining in your mouth. How long does it last?

Now think a bit about how you usually eat. I'm not suggesting that you should do all your eating the way you just ate your grape; lunch breaks just aren't long enough. But I will suggest that you apply something of this mindfulness to your patterns of eating.

When you eat, do you usually do something else at the same time? My own tendency is to grab something to read while I eat. Do you read or watch TV while you eat?

Do you ever eat an entire meal or snack without really noticing what you're eating? It's quite possible to eat three full meals a day on automatic pilot. If you're not paying attention to the act of eating itself, what are you paying attention to?

How long does it take you to eat each meal? I've seen my extended family demolish a complete turkey dinner with all the trimmings, including dessert, in less than an hour. Would you classify yourself as a fast eater, a slow eater, or in between? Are you a nibbler or a gulper? How long would it normally take you to eat a donut?

Remember that we're talking about mindfulness here. I recommend that you not try to change your food habits very much at the beginning. Just pay attention. Again, if it helps your mindfulness of your food habits to write them down, go for it.

In the last chapter on weight management, I didn't ask you to change anything about your food intake. Nor am I here. If there's some small thing you've noticed that you think is counter-productive in terms of the way you would like to operate, and you specifically want to change it, go ahead. But the important thing at this point is not so much what you change, but to pay attention to

how that change affects how you think and feel.

Let's say you've noticed that your usual pattern is to be almost totally oblivious of what you're eating, because your attention is on TV or a book or magazine. You might decide that before you turn on the TV or pick up the book, you'll eat a bite or two something like the way you ate that grape. That's good. It's an experiment. Notice what happens. Notice what your mind does with this. Notice whether this approach becomes a habit that you continue to practice, or whether after a day or two or a week or two you revert to your previous approach.

One more thing about mindfulness and food. One of the books I list at the end of the book refers to some types of food as "bait." This is food that we are inclined to eat not because we're particularly hungry or need nourishment, but because it tastes so good. Think of the difference between a tasty bowl of lentil curry with a piece of whole wheat bread and a box of chocolate-covered macadamia nuts. We'll get into the distinction between healthy and not-so-healthy foods later, but for now pay a little attention to your eating throughout the day in terms of "food" vs. "bait."

We're not quite done with the mouth yet.

If you can't control what goes into your mouth, what can you control?

If you can't control what comes out of your mouth, what can you control?

These two questions are somewhat facile and misleading. They imply that controlling what goes into and comes out of the mouth represents a basic or low level of control. On the contrary, controlling those two things relates to core functions of skillful living: that is, living in such a way as to move from pain and unhappiness toward happiness and richness of life.

In the tradition of Vipassana meditation, there is a two-way street between meditation proper and right living. Meditation and the knowledge of reality move the meditator in the direction of right living. Right living, in turn, supports the quest for insight or wisdom as well as happiness.

There are five specific rules or precepts for life, corresponding in some ways to the ten commandments of the Judeo-Christian tradition. Here they are:

- ✓ Don't kill or use violence against other sentient beings;
- ✓ Don't steal, or take what's not freely given;
- ✓ Don't engage in sexual misconduct: i.e., don't use sexual energy in a way that causes harm;
- ✓ Don't lie, use harsh or idle speech, or harm others through speech;
- ✓ Don't use intoxicants to befuddle your mind and cause heedlessness.

Notice that two of the precepts relate to the mouth. The precept about lying relates to all harmful uses of words. The last precept relates to any kind of addictive or unhealthy use of consumables, including food.

In addition, you may have noticed earlier in this chapter that Skillful Speech is Step 3 of the Eightfold Path to happiness.

So far we've just been talking about mindfulness with regard to food and eating. Now I'm suggesting that you extend your mindfulness not only to what goes into your mouth, but to what comes out of your mouth as well.

The four parts of Skillful Speech in the Vipassana tradition are

> ➢ Tell the truth;
> ➢ Avoid malicious talk;
> ➢ Speak gently and kindly, avoiding abusive, sarcastic, or critical speech;
> ➢ Avoid idle or useless chatter.

This chapter has introduced a new level of issues. A person could work on them for many years. There's a danger here: to begin to feel overwhelmed or discouraged at the realization of how profoundly one might need to change simply in order to manage skillfully what goes into and comes out of the mouth.

Be gentle with yourself. As you become more mindful of the mouth, you're not more out of control than you've been in the past. You're just becoming more aware of what's going on in this area, and how central it might be to an overall skillful and healthy life.

Try to barely notice your habits and patterns of the mouth: what goes in and what comes out. Avoid being judgmental or critical of yourself.

Meditators say the most important moment in your meditation is when you get up off your zafu and go about the rest of your day. Mindfulness if not for meditation; meditation and mindfulness are for life. They are ways to access the Eightfold Path that leads from the "normal" suffering of human life to a satisfying happiness through skillful practices.

In the next chapter we'll go into an important issue directly involving both what goes into the mouth and what comes out of it: the issue of talking about your new weight management method with other people. Before you read that chapter, think a bit about what your tendency might be. Are you inclined to process things like this verbally with family or friends? Or are you more inclined to keep what you're doing to yourself? Why do you think you do whichever you do?

Mindful Message: Pain is inevitable; suffering is optional. As you learn that the ego is not you, you can also learn to observe occurrences in the body like pain, hunger, craving, anxiety, or restlessness with an objective attitude that acknowledges pain without inducing suffering. What would hunger or craving for a particular food item feel like in the absence of judgment, aversion, desire, or a feeling of obligation to do something about it? You can find this out for yourself.

VI. GETTING INTO THE GROOVE

Remember Chapter IV? In the example, our 162 pound person decided that if she continued as in the past, in three months she would weigh 163.5 pounds. She set the apparently modest goal of weighing 159 pounds at the end of that three month period, losing one pound per month.

What was your beginning weight, and what did you set as your goal? Did you write both of them down? Have you continued to weigh yourself and write down your weight every morning since?

For many people, it is easier to accomplish such a goal by the middle of next week than it is to reach the same goal by the end of three months. For many of us, a few days of starvation is easier than three months of deliberate mindfulness and small changes.

There are a number of good reasons for this. We can do anything as long as it's for just a short time. But permanent changes in our life routines are more difficult. More about this in the next chapter.

One thing I've noticed in my own practice is that my intentions have to be very specific and clear. My monkey mind is cunning and manipulative, especially in the area of food and weight. It will contrive to cause itself as little inconvenience as possible compatible with meeting the minimum requirements I set.

Do you notice in this last paragraph how I am deliberately not identifying with "my" monkey mind or ego? One of the products of mindfulness is to be able to distinguish between the monkey mind and something else in myself that is aware of or mindful of the monkey mind.

This business about intentionality is critical. Let me give you an example so this is as clear as possible.

I originally set my intention to reduce my weight to 175 pounds and to maintain it there. The first day I saw the number 175 (actually 175.6) on my scale, I believed I had reduced my weight to 175 pounds.

Now I had to consider: What does it mean to maintain my weight at this new level? Does it mean that every day my weight has to be 175 or less? How do I accommodate the natural tendency of weight to vary a pound or two from day to day?

I decided that weighing 175 was compatible with allowing two pounds of variance. Any number on my scale between 173 and 177 was OK.

As I continued to weigh myself each morning and record my weight, I noticed something odd: I never saw the number 173. I never saw the number 174. And I rarely saw the number 175. My weight was consistently either 176 or 177 point something.

Because I had gotten so good at controlling my weight within a narrow variance, when the number threatened to exceed the upper limit of 177 I could keep it from slipping over 177 into the 178 level. But because I had created some flexibility in my intention, my monkey mind took full advantage of the flexibility: it turned out that I had reduced my weight not to 175 but to 177, the upper limit of the allowable.

This is the nature of the monkey mind. It is cunning and it is a manipulator. It is a subtle game-player. That's why it is so important not only to set an intention, but also to define the intention precisely. Reduce the ambiguity as much as possible.

So let's get much more specific about the goal of our Example Person (EP). Does weighing one pound less in one month mean that sometime between now and one month from now I will on at least one occasion weigh 161 pounds instead of my initial weight of 162? This is clearly not specific enough. The objective is that one month from now, I will weigh not 0.5 pounds more than I weigh now, but one pound less. Further, EP is already projecting beyond the first month and anticipating that in three months, instead of weighing 163.5 she will weigh 159.

Go a step further. Have you noticed how your weight fluctuates from day to day, and how today's results aren't always responsive to what went into your mouth yesterday? Have you figured out why this is? I imagine you've noticed that your pattern of bowel movements has something to do with your weight on any particular morning. Maybe you've noticed some relationship to salt intake and fluid retention. Maybe you've noticed some variance around your menstrual cycle. Is there anything else you've observed that results in fluctuations of a few pounds in your weight?

Go back and look at the numbers you've posted for the last three full weeks. What's the difference in each of those weeks between the highest number and the lowest number? You can probably expect about that much variance to continue, even as your average weight declines. So you need to program that phenomenon of variation into your intention-setting.

When I noticed that the way I had defined weighing 175 pounds had resulted in a process where I was succeeding in meeting my goals even though I might never actually see the number 175 on my scale, I decided that I would redefine my goal or intention. In my new definition, I would be successful only if at least once each week I did in fact see the number 175 on my scale.

Now that you're familiar with the cunning manipulation of the monkey mind, I'll bet you can predict what happened next. Yes, my records show that I was now managing my weight in such a way that once each week I was seeing the number 175 on my scale. The other six days of the week I would see either 176 or 177, and even an occasional 178.

Maybe that's OK. As long as I see 175 once a week, my weight is pretty successfully anchored at an acceptable level. But that seems a very grudging approach to what I'm trying to accomplish. When I look back over my calendar and see a week or two during which the lowest recorded weight is 175.8, it doesn't make me feel good. But if I look at two weeks later, I see the following readings: 176.4; 175.0; 174.6; 174.6; 174.8; 175.0; 175.8. That makes me feel much better. So while I haven't formulated a new intention yet, I probably will create one that reflects something closer to that performance.

Intention is powerful, but it must also be specific and focused.

For EP, let's set our goal quite specifically. Her program started on Monday, November 4, 2013. Since we're keeping track of weeks from Monday morning through Sunday night, let's create 28 day months for convenience. Sunday, December 1, 2013 will be the end of the first month and December 2 will be the beginning of the second for EP's program. So let's set the goal that on the seven days starting December 1, EP's weight should not exceed 161 (161 includes any of the decimals of 161 from 161.0 to 161.9) on more than two of those seven days.

Looking forward three months, we'll do the same thing. January 27, 2014 will be the first day of the fourth month of EP's program. To be successful at that point, during the week starting January 27 her weight can exceed 159 on no more than two days.

Once the goal has been set and clearly articulated, you'll begin to see that there will be plenty to manage in the weeks leading up to the final week of each month. You might decide that it would be prudent to make sure you have come very close to that goal the preceding week.

And here we first encounter one of the key concepts of the Mindfulness Method of Weight Management. Once you set your goal and focus your intention, you have infinite flexibility in how you choose to accomplish the goal. The only firm requirements are that you weigh yourself each morning and record your weight; and that you continue to practice regular mindfulness meditation at least at the minimum level described in the last chapter, hopefully building up to a total of twenty minutes a day by the end of the first three month period. Beyond that, how you manage to meet your goal is entirely up to you. The remaining chapters in this book are all about creating a framework of mindfulness in meditation and in weight management to help you with that process.

If you decided that, since you have a whole month to achieve your goal of losing one pound, you'll devote the first week to eating everything in sight, you will see, at least once a day, the results of that decision. You will learn something during that week, and you will be experiencing certain feelings and thoughts related to that decision. Just pay attention.

Or you might have decided that you would experiment during the first week of the one month period to see what it would take in terms of your food intake to register 161 on your scale at least one day of that week. Just pay attention to what happens and what you feel and think about what happens. You're practicing mindfulness.

Did you notice what just changed? Before you were only asked to observe. Now you are now being asked to change something about your food intake, **and** to observe and record the results. What you change is up to you. But you are now for the first time applying the three core requirements of the system of Mindfulness and Weight Management:

- Make a mindful change in your food patterns;

- Pay attention to how that change affects the message your scale gives you;

- Pay attention to how both the change in your food patterns and the message from your scale affect your feelings and thoughts.

Just pay attention, and see what this experiment produces.

As you play with making changes to your food habits and mindfully observing the results, it might be interesting to go back to Chapter II where I asked you to start paying attention to eating patterns. Review what you noticed, and consider looking at some of the patterns you identified for possible experimentation.

Let's say you noticed a pattern of snacking during the two hours prior to your usual bedtime of 11:00. Your snacks usually consisted of sweets, the most usual being half a dozen cookies or a quarter of a pint of ice cream. You could experiment during the first week with substituting something with less calories, or perhaps eating half as much but eating it very slowly and mindfully.

Or maybe a pattern was keeping a bag of your favorite mini-size candy bars in your desk, and having one or two each time you get a cup of coffee or tea during the day. You might experiment with substituting something with half the calories, or joining a friend or co-worker to chat over tea or coffee instead of snacking at your desk.

Make a change. Be mindful of how it feels. Pay attention to the results.

If you are used to standard diet programs, this may seem very open-ended and unclear at this point. Don't worry. You're resourceful and intelligent, and you've got a framework that allows you to find solutions day by day that are just right for you. Your issues (the myriad of factors that have produced a person with exactly your weight, height, complexion, set of ideas, modes of feelings, etc) are not identical to anybody else's. What happens to you when you meditate isn't identical to what happens to anybody else. As I mentioned, the rest of this book will flesh out the outline provided so far and give you plenty of additional guidance on how to proceed.

Now let's switch gears and open another topic.

So far we've not talked about the quality of food at all, only its calorie content. There are some reasons for that.

You can follow every piece of advice or instruction in this book and learn to manage your weight successfully while eating an absolutely atrocious diet and creating all sorts of health issues for yourself. I hope you won't do that. But I want you to be completely clear that healthy eating and weight control are two related but separate issues.

Confusing the two can cause problems in both. Some popular diets are popular because they promise that you can eat as much as you want of specific foods or types of food. Some promote the idea that if you eat only "healthy foods" you will reach and maintain your ideal weight.

Your relative consumption of carbohydrates and fats and protein and fiber is important. Whether you are a vegetarian or a vegan or an omnivore is important. But you can gain weight or lose weight with any combination of foods in your diet.

A tablespoon of oil contains about 120 calories, all from fat. That's almost as many calories as a whole can of Coke. Oils tend to contain at least three types of fat: saturated fat, polyunsaturated fat, and mono-unsaturated fat. Does it matter what types of oil you use and the percentages of the different types of fat? Sure it does. Some are healthier than others. But if you consume eight tablespoons full of the healthiest oil on the market, you will still have taken in almost a thousand calories.

What would that do to your weight? How would it make you feel? One result that's pretty predictable is that if you only consumed 2000 calories today, and half of that consisted of 8 tablespoons of high quality olive oil, you would probably feel hungry. The calorie content of something doesn't have much connection to its mass or weight and the feeling of fullness it gives you.

The nice thing is that most of us aren't tempted to take little sips of vegetable oil throughout the day. We like to get our fat mixed in with other things, particularly spices and sugars. Remember the distinction between bait and food? If something is a particularly successful bait, you can bet it's loaded with at least two out of three of those ingredients: fat, spices, and sugar.

You can lose weight on a diet of nothing but bacon cheeseburgers and fries. You just can't eat very many of them. Try it if you want to. What does it do to your weight? How does it make you feel?

Try anything you want to. What does it do to the message your scale gives you? How does it make you feel? Make a decision, act on it, then pay attention to the results. Experiment.

When you grocery shop, do you read labels?

How much do you know about the food industry in your country? Have you read any books or articles about how food is processed and marketed?

Is most of the food you buy and consume processed and packaged? How much of it is at the bottom end of the food chain: beans, rice, lentils; fresh fruits; fresh vegetables?

Is there a farmers' market near you? Have you checked it out? Do you see any value in supporting local food production and marketing?

Do you own any cookbooks? What type?

Just as your bathroom scale is a mindfulness tool related to weight management, the things mentioned above are all related to mindfulness of one type of another about food. It's not necessary for you to be or to become an expert on nutrition, but you probably will find that some basic information about foods and food preparation is an aid to food mindfulness.

I find it much more pleasant and easy to maintain the weight I choose if I have a good supply of healthy, nutritious foods around. I've learned to make some breads that are much tastier and healthier than anything I can find to buy. I can make a walnut/lentil loaf that's great for lunches, and a rice pudding that's perfect for snacks. And I can modestly claim that my cinnamon rolls, when they first come out of the oven, are fabulous. I've provided a few recipes in Appendix B in case you want to try any of these things.

Cooking and baking simple healthy meals is a wonderful exercise in mindfulness. When I bake my cranraison/pecan bread, I'll use five or six different kinds of flour instead of sticking with the basic processed or bleached wheat flour. Each has a slightly different look and feel, and I've read that barley and oat flour, for example, have different micro-nutrients than wheat flour. I like to throw in a little wheat germ and some flax seed meal. I usually substitute some cooked steel-cut oats or left over potatoes or rice or couscous for some of the flour. I've found that adding a hefty dose of cinnamon makes the experience of toasting this bread for breakfast an olfactory delight.

Maybe you don't have the time or inclination to do much cooking or baking. I suggest that if you don't currently do any, or very little, you try just one or two items. Prepare them with care and attention. Take a little extra time eating them. Pay attention to how making something particularly tasty and healthy makes you feel, and whether you find any special pleasure in preparing and eating it and sharing it with friends or family.

My cinnamon rolls, cranraison/pecan bread, and omelets have become family legends already, and I get a lot of pleasure from filling special requests from visiting family and friends.

This is a big chapter, but I still need to connect your food management with what comes out of your mouth, as promised in the last chapter.

I've decided against making a recommendation as to whether you should discuss this weight management method with other people. My inclination is to recommend against, but how much is that just my own preferences or personality type speaking? What seems best to me may be a disaster for you. So instead of making a recommendation, I'll just give you some guidelines for thinking about this and making a conscious decision about it.

First, the positive side. There is such a thing as community. Meditators call it the "sangha;" Christians call it the church. The purpose of community is to support an individual in, hopefully, improving conduct of life and increasing happiness.

Many people find this kind of organized support essential. Some diet programs and smoking cessation programs make this support an integral part of their approach. You talk about what you're trying to do in your life, and your community supports you at least in the positive or accepted parts of your attempts at improvement.

Sharing your goals and plans doesn't have to be that organized. Most people have at least one or two people in their lives they count on for sharing and support. Some people can't imagine going into a new method of weight management without talking it over with one or more of those people, and it would be unthinkable not to give them a blow by blow account of how it's going. Talking about what you are doing, for many people, is a way of making it more real, and getting encouragement, praise, or some other form of support helps focus the attention on maintaining the program.

If this sounds right for you, try it. But before you decide to talk about your new program, consider the following points.

Too often, talking is a substitute for action. It's possible, after "talking through" an idea, to feel that we've disposed of it. I hear people talking endlessly about their diets and diet failures, and I don't see much relationship between the amount of verbal attention something gets and the meaningful action or practical results. Think about exactly what it is you need or expect to get by talking to someone about this attempt.

Talking is very random and unorganized. There's a reason I took five and a half chapters before asking you to change anything significant about your eating patterns. It's necessary to lay some groundwork, and to make sure you are practicing at least the rudiments of a mindfulness program before you tackle diet changes. When you tell your friend about this program, you might say: "I'm reading this book about meditation and weight. The guy says just to start meditating and weighing yourself every day, and your whole relationship to food and your body will automatically begin to change." What's your friend supposed to say: "Wow! That sounds great; I'll bet it works for you." More likely the underlying message will be something like: "Don't get sucked into some weird cultish approach to eating. By the way, I know somebody who took Supplement X and lost 50 pounds."

Finally, consider an intermediate approach. Consider keeping your own counsel while you give this method your serious commitment for three months. Don't talk to anybody not only about the mindfulness method but about the various choices you're making as you implement it. There's no real need to mention to anyone that you've reduced your canned drinks from three a day to one. Instead of talking to someone about your thoughts and feelings as you go along, meditate about them or keep a diary or journal. Focus the energy inward instead of outward.

If you are successfully working the mindfulness method, you can be pretty sure that at some point, after maybe three months or six months, people will start saying things to you about the changes they observe. Women in particular are uncannily observant. My wife and I know a couple where the man is easily 100 pounds overweight. One evening my wife commented to him that he looked like he had lost some weight. I couldn't see any difference at all. It turned out that he had made a bet with a friend about who could lose the most weight in two weeks. He had lost five pounds (and easily won the bet). Once you start getting comments, it's fine to say: "Thank you. I've been trying a completely different approach to managing my weight, and so far I'm very happy." If they're truly interested, you can lend them your book.

At a minimum, don't be totally casual about the issue of talking about your program. Decide in advance who you will discuss it with, and think about what you think you will gain by doing so. Keep in mind that this program is absolutely for you. As you progress, you are the one who will feel and see the difference, and your own satisfaction is what you are after. You are developing more skillful methods of living your life. You are reducing the unsatisfactory parts of your life in a targeted way and increasing your satisfaction or happiness.

You have now initiated a cycle that's going to become very familiar to you. You observe a pattern. You make a decision to change something about the pattern, and do it. You pay attention to the results: how it makes you feel; what you think about it; what your scales tell you.

You avoid getting judgmental with yourself as you do this. You pay attention to how the results relate to the goals you've set for yourself this day or this week. You use yesterday's and last week's results to set your intention for tomorrow or for next week. You're in the groove.

Mindful Message: Too often, talking about something in a substitute for taking meaningful action about it.   Make a conscious decision about whether and how much and to whom you will talk about your weight management issues.   Focus on getting positive results for yourself for your own reasons.   It's OK to just let others notice and comment on your results.

VII. ATTACHMENT, HABITS, AND CHANGE

In the Vipassana meditation tradition, there's a lot of focus on attachment. That's because attachment is considered to be the root of human suffering. In the practice of mindfulness meditation, and in the application of mindfulness to weight management, one of the things we're pretty sure to run into is the way attachments dominate our lives.

Attachment has two sides: wanting something; and wanting to avoid something. Wanting comfort and ease is the flip side of wanting to avoid discomfort. Wanting to be with someone is the flip side of wanting to avoid contact with someone.

Human beings, seen from the inside, as happens in meditation, can appear to be nothing more than bundles of attachments. We can operate like behavioral toys, now attracted by this and that, now repelled by other things.

Habits are more or less fixed patterns of feelings and actions based on attachments. We act in certain ways based on our attachment to certain results. For example, if we're hungry we might think about food, evaluate possible sources of food, make decisions based on that evaluation, and then act on the decisions.

It's also possible that we might go through the pattern of action described in the last paragraph not because we're hungry, but because it's noon and we're in the habit of eating lunch at noon. The pattern of action is triggered not by a certain feeling in our bodies but by the clock.

The part of this description I would like you to focus on is this: habits are "patterns of feelings and actions." Typically, habits are expressed in processes that follow those patterns more or less automatically. Habits tend to be not single actions, but patterned sequences of actions, or processes.

I'll give an example of a "pattern of feelings and action" from personal relationships, not weight management, just to show how broadly this concept applies.

If you're in a long term relationship, it's probably safe to say that there are things your partner does that push your buttons. It could be a certain kind of criticism. Maybe a habitual comment about your appearance. Maybe a habit of being late for appointments. Human beings typically have dozens if not hundreds of buttons of this type.

What happens when a button is pushed? Most likely it triggers a habitual pattern of feelings and actions. Let me give an example I'm very familiar with.

My wife and I are planning to go out to play bridge at a bridge club. The games start precisely at the scheduled time, and once the game starts, new arrivals can't be added. The location of the particular game we're going to is about 30 minutes away when traffic is normal. I'm ready to go, and have been for fifteen minutes, and I'm waiting for my wife to finish her preparations. It's 40 minutes to game time. Then it's 35 minutes to game time. I like to be early to games, as my wife is aware. At

32 minutes to game time I go to the bedroom and say "Are you ready to go? We're going to be late." My wife says "I'll be right there." Three minutes later she's ready to go. I'm tense and angry that she's once again set us up to have to rush and get to the game at the last minute. She's casual and relaxed and makes some inconsequential comment as we pull out of the driveway. I don't answer. She glances at me and notices my set jaw. A predictable conversation begins, and goes through its predictable course to its predictable conclusion.

Do you have scripted patterns like this? Have you identified habits or patterns like this that you would like to change, but haven't been able to?

What I recommend you do for starters is to begin to pay attention to habits you may have around food. Be grateful that this isn't a book about personal relationships; then you'd have to dive right in to the really tough habits. Food is easier.

What patterns of feelings and actions do you have around food?

Mindfulness is your tool; it's your way to turn off the automatic pilot and examine how things work. What's odd about us human beings is that we are typically more mindful of the habits of other people than about our own. It's much easier to observe the habits of others and maybe even to understand them. Why? Because of attachment. We have a very heavy vested interest in protecting our own habits, and our egos are adept at helping us ignore or justify them.

This habit of not being mindful of our own patterns of feelings and actions can be a great disservice to our true interests if, for example, our interest is in changing some habit.

Vipassana meditation manuals talk a lot about the dhamma (sometimes called the dharma), which has several layers of meaning. One meaning is "the way things are," or "the nature of things," or just "reality." A second meaning is "the way we need to be in order to live in alignment with the way things are." If things are a certain way, but we act as if they were some other way, the universe is likely to give us negative feedback. If we think weight management is about having a positive self-image, but it's really about calory intake, working on a positive self-image while consuming a pint of ice cream on a regular basis will produce results we won't like.

But don't get the idea that a positive self-image, or self-esteem, isn't relevant to weight management. It's so important that much of Chapter XI is devoted to it. Self-esteem is very often critically misunderstood in our society.

Understanding "the way things are" is a prerequisite to changing what is.

So pay attention to your "dhamma of food." What is it with you and food? What are your patterns of feelings and actions around food? Make them explicit. Remember intentionality, and the importance of being specific in terms of what your intentions are? This is another place where specificity is important. Take notes. Write descriptions of what you notice. What do you want? What do you crave? What don't you like? How do you react to your feelings about food? How does eating or not eating make you feel?

Among other things, pay attention to what it feels like to be hungry. Many of us, much of the time, don't ever go without food long enough to experience that feeling. Give yourself a chance to feel it, and pay attention to how it feels. See if you can tell the difference between "being hungry" and "wanting to eat something."

When you notice something you might categorize as a "habit about food," write it down and see if you can break it down into steps of a process. Let me give you an example.

Once a week you attend a social function that lasts about three hours, from 2:00 to 5:00. At this function, snacks and treats are always available. When you're watching your weight, or trying to lose a few pounds, or dieting, this function can be quite a trial to you. You've noticed that you are already thinking about the food before you get to the event. You're determined not to be thrown off your diet by some tempting sweet, but you're more or less constantly aware of the food. Everybody else is having some, and people will say to you: "These chocolate covered macadamia nuts are incredible. Have you tried them?" "I just can't stay away from that dip. Here, try a little."

Whether you end up having something or not, the afternoon is miserable for you. And what's the point? Your attempts to be disciplined don't seem to have any significant or lasting positive results anyway.

This is a situation around which you are exercising a habit, a pattern of feelings and actions. Write it down in detail. Notice whether or not you say anything about your struggle to any of the other participants. If you do, what do you say? How many times in the course of the afternoon do you mention the food or your attempts to avoid eating it? How do you feel if you tough it out and don't eat a single morsel? How do you feel if you give in and have something?

Another example. You tend to have a light dinner, which you've usually finished by about 7:00. You've read that it's not a good idea to eat much late in the evening close to bed time. The problem is that you've developed the habit of having a late dessert, not a lot, but something sweet. If you don't, you'll find yourself recurrently thinking about it all evening. Generally, even if you're trying to cut back on evening snacks, your resistance will be worn down over the course of several hours, and you'll find something to satisfy that hunger.

Most of us can identify half a dozen habits or patterns like these two around food pretty easily. See if you can. Pay attention to them, and write them down in detail if you can. It may help you identify these patterns by thinking in terms of each of the three standard meals, plus eating between meals.

These habits related to food are part of your food dhamma. They are part of the way things are. They are part of your way of relating to the way things are.

By now you've probably noticed a (possibly annoying) habit of mine in this book. I'll tell you to notice something, to pay attention to it, to be mindful of it, and then I'll recommend that you not do anything immediately to try to change it.

What happens when I do that? How do you feel about it? How does it feel to be mindful of a habit, especially of a "bad" habit, and not try to do anything to change it? Pay attention to that feeling, as well as to any actions you are inclined to take in response to that feeling.

As you pursue your meditation, you'll get more familiar with attachment. In time you'll start becoming aware of habits that grow out of various kinds of attachment. You'll suddenly notice (become mindful of) yourself in one or another step of a process that springs with great predictability from a particular attachment.

Now if all your habits are "good" habits, you can stop here. However, if any of your habits, especially habits related to food, could use some slight changes, you'll need to keep going. This chapter is about attachment, habits, and change; those three things go together. We've covered the first two, but we'll defer our detailed look at change until after we take care of a couple of other related issues in the next few chapters.

For now, just focus on identifying and describing your food habits. Try to see how the habits are made up of processes, and notice if you can how an attachment or desire or repulsion is at the root of the habit.

Mindful Message: Understanding the way things are is a pre-requisite to changing the parts of your current reality that don't serve you well: i.e., habits that are not skillful.

In the middle of Chapter VI, we finally got around to asking you to make some changes in your eating patterns and to pay attention to what happened. Let's say you've been applying the three core steps of the mindfulness method of weight management for two weeks. I'm sure you remember what they are, but let's make sure:

- Making a mindful change in your food patterns;

- Paying attention to how that change affects the message your scale gives you each morning;

- Paying attention to how both the change in your food patterns and the message from your scale affect your feelings and thoughts.

Now let's apply this to Example Person (EP). Remember her? She decided that her goal for the first three months of her new program was to weigh 159 pounds instead of the 163.5 she was headed toward by the end of three months. A deeper goal was to use that first three month period to establish some habits that would begin to put her in control of her weight.

On Monday of the first week of her program, EP weighed 162 pounds. She decided that she would use the first two weeks of the three months experimenting with some of the techniques she had been reading about. She would change something specific about her eating patterns, and she would pay attention to what happened as a result. She would notice what message her scale would give her day by day; how she would feel about the changes in her eating patterns; and how she would feel about the scale's messages.

One of the patterns EP had noticed was one she shared with millions of other Americans. Her favorite beverage was soft drinks, particularly Coke. As part of her attempt to be more mindful about what she put in her mouth, she read the ingredients list on the Coke can. She observed that the two main ingredients of Coke are carbonated water and high fructose corn syrup. A can of Coke contains no fat, which she thought was a mark in its favor, but it also contains no protein, and all the carbohydrate content was from the 39 grams of sugar in each can. She also noticed that each can has 140 calories. She knew from an article she had read that these are what are called "empty calories," meaning they have no value in terms of basic nourishment. As an afterthought she made a note of the fact that each gram of sugar is the equivalent of about 3 ½ calories.

It didn't take EP long to figure out that 140 calories was 7% of the 2000 calories she estimated she needed each day to maintain a constant weight. And she had observed as she paid attention to her food patterns that she typically would drink two Cokes per day, sometimes three. When she learned that consuming 3600 calories was the equivalent of adding a pound of weight, she did the math (140 X 2 X 30 = 8400 calories per month) and figured out that at the rate of two Cokes per day, she was adding a little over two pounds per month.

"What would it feel like," EP asked herself, "if I were to limit myself to one Coke per day for a while. I wonder if that would show up on my scale." She decided she would consider this pattern change as her initial experiment.

As she thought about it, she wondered how she could hold everything else about her eating constant. How would she know whether she was adding calories somewhere else in her daily eating?

She decided that in addition to holding her Coke intake to one can per day, she would simply pay attention to her eating, being on the lookout for simple and non-painful ways to keep her calory intake under control. And each time she was mindful of deliberately having less of something than she might have taken in the past, she would pay attention to how it felt and would notice whether it affected the messages her bathroom scale gave her.

When you make your first decision to change something about your food habits, and then you observe what happens, there are three primary possibilities. One, you might notice some changes you consider positive. Two, you might notice some changes you consider negative. Three, your observed results might be neutral or ambiguous.

EP found the first two weeks quite interesting. One thing she continued to notice about her formal meditation practice was that her sessions seemed to fall into two categories. She was able on some days to focus pretty successfully on her breathing and to feel her body and her monkey mind calming down and relaxing. On other days, she could hardly manage in her 10-15 minute sessions to actually keep track of a single breath from beginning to end without her mind racing off on some tangent.

She was able to accept that both were OK, though she did feel some frustration on the days she couldn't get to that peaceful inward space she was beginning to recognize and want more of.

As for the "food dhamma," she was fascinated to notice how little connection there was between even mild hunger and the desire to eat. One thing in particular she noticed was the compulsion to finish whatever was in front of her, without regard to how full or empty she felt. Slowing down the process of eating as well as eating several times a week without the distraction of TV or reading helped her with a key observation: if she filled her plate with lots of food, she automatically continued to eat until the plate was empty. If she put less on her plate, she didn't feel inclined to add more after she had cleaned her plate.

Sometimes she would become aware that she was full before her plate was empty, but force of habit inclined her strongly to keep eating until all the food was gone. She realized she could almost hear her mother's voice saying "Waste not, want not," and she remembered when she was growing up her mother's satisfaction when she was "a member of the Clean Plate Club."

She had used this insight to alter a key early step in the process she had identified. When she was filling her plate or setting out the food she intended to eat, she would deliberately give herself adequate but not excessive portions. She felt that this had allowed her to cut back her calorie intake to some extent without any pain or even discomfort.

After your first two weeks of practice of mindfulness and weight management, you could write a similar little story. If you think it would be helpful to keep some sort of record or notes, go for it. **If you do, you might find, as many others have, that writing and thinking about what you've done can lead you to helpful insights that you might have missed otherwise.** One reason for this is that writing forces you to slow down; it almost forces the writer to pay more, or a different kind of, attention to the experience.

Now let's go back to the three possible results EP (and you) might have experienced: positive; negative; ambiguous. Here are the recorded weights reflecting each experience for the two week period.

	Positive		Negative
Ambiguous			
Monday	162.0	162.0	162.0
Tuesday	162.8	162.2	162.8
Wednesday	162.2	162.2	162.8
Thursday	161.9	162.8	162.4
Friday	162.0	163.1	162.8
Saturday	161.6	162.7	162.0
Sunday	161.7	163.2	163.0

Monday	161.6	162.9	162.4
Tuesday	162.1	163.3	162.0
Wednesday	161.6	163.0	161.8
Thursday	161.4	163.2	162.2
Friday	161.9	163.4	161.8
Saturday	161.2	163.4	162.6
Sunday	160.9	163.0	161.6

In the first scenario, you notice that the number 162 becomes more and more rare, and lower numbers start to take over. That's good; your intention is that very soon you will never again see the number 162 or any higher number on your scale.

In the second scenario, the opposite happened. Whatever you've chosen to do during the first two weeks, the message from your scale is that it's not working. Not only is your weight not trending slowly downward; you appear to have gained a pound in spite of your efforts.

In the third scenario, your weight is still 162 or over four out of seven days in the second week. Not terrible, but not what you would prefer to see.

What's important about these scenarios? The most important thing is how you feel about this information and what you do with it.

Some weight management gurus think it's a big mistake to weigh yourself so often. Some think you shouldn't weigh yourself at all. To them, it's just a way of enslaving yourself to a system that doesn't recognize the true measure of your success: how you perceive yourself and how you feel about yourself. In their view, you shouldn't measure success in terms of meeting somebody else's idea of what your "correct" weight is.

In the system I'm laying out in this book, weighing yourself every day is important, but it's what you do with the data that's truly important. That's why I've created these three scenarios, each of which will match some reader's experience after two weeks of working this program. Let's talk about what you can do with whichever scenario fits your experience.

If you have approached the first two weeks like EP did, the most likely and most realistic result is the positive scenario. The results may quite likely be even more positive than you expected. The initial enthusiasm you might feel for your new program is likely to make you extra conscientious about both your meditation and your eating. It may well be that the main thing you have to do with your first two weeks' results is to cool it a little. It's tempting to think: "Hey, this is a piece of cake. I'll bet I can drop two pounds next week. I was way too modest in setting my three-month goal."

One of the four primary personal characteristics that meditation supports and nourishes is equanimity, or emotional balance. The typical reaction to positive results by a person with equanimity might be simply to register the results of the experiment, to notice the satisfaction that is a logical response to positive results, and to think about whether any changes are called for going into the next two week period.

Fast weight loss is frequently the kiss of death. Slow, incremental, consistent loss is the key to long term success in weight management. If you have already reached your three month goal after two weeks, be very careful. **Don't change your three month goal.** That doesn't mean you should go out of your way not to exceed your three month goal. You should consolidate what you have learned during the first two weeks, decide whether to continue your food management behavior without change as you go into week three or whether to change it in some way, and continue to act, observe results, and pay attention.

This is so important I want to risk being repetitious. If you goal was to lose one pound per month for the first three months, and after three weeks you have already gone from 162 to 159, **you have not met your goal.** Many, many people can lose three pounds in three weeks, but not in three months! There is no basis for exuberance here. Simply note what you're seeing on your scale, notice how it makes you feel and think; and then soberly decide what your strategy will be for the next week.

What if you have the Negative scenario? You have made some changes that you expected to produce positive results, and instead your lying, rotten scale persists in telling you you've gained a solid pound more than you started with.

There are several things you could do in response. Despair is not the recommended option. You have conducted an experiment, and the results were surprising and disappointing.

First, go back over your two weeks as objectively as you can. Were there any days you actually had two Cokes instead of the one you decided on? Did you ever notice during the two week period that you took opportunities to supplement your food intake in ways you hadn't planned? Any special parties or events where you pigged out? Any evening food binges?

Can you identify any anomalies in your eating during the two weeks that might explain the failure to see any lower weights? Or are the results totally perplexing and irrational?

Don't panic. If you feel after thoughtful review that your calorie intake absolutely was consistently lower than normal, and you still didn't see any positive results, there are a couple of options you have.

The first is to continue as before. Simply continue to apply the changes you made during the first two weeks and see is the results change. They might. Weight management can be pretty idiosyncratic. I've had weeks when my weight seemed absolutely unmovable and unresponsive to anything I might do. Then the next week, the low numbers would pop up on my scale like a delayed reaction. Continue to observe your patterns, notice what you are doing, how it feels, what the results are.

The second thing you might try is to make additional changes. I recommend against getting too stringent with yourself based on any short term results or lack of results. But maybe you've noticed that you don't miss the second Coke at all, and drinking water, tea, or coffee feels OK. So maybe you drop the Coke altogether for the next two weeks. But be careful not to over-react.

A third possibility is a special measure to guard against the natural tendency we have to deceive ourselves about food and drink. (That tendency, by the way, is one reason we use the scale daily to give us objective feedback about our weight.)

I knew someone who was chronically overweight who would visit my wife and me regularly and who invariably would talk about how she had had nothing to eat all day except a couple of carrot sticks. In the course of a couple of hours, an enormous number of calories would disappear into her mouth, and it was clear that she had very limited awareness that this was happening. To her, it was totally inexplicable that she continued to gain weight.

Some people find a food diary very helpful as an aid to mindfulness. This should be something you carry with you all day so you can whip it out every time you put anything into your mouth, even a single potato chip. (As if any of us can eat just one.) Sometime people are astonished at the things they find recorded in their food diary after a day. Of course it's easy to forget or omit things, but as your mindfulness increases, you'll remember to jot down "Cookie from Anna, 10:45 am," and "Coffee break; 2 pm, pastry with coffee." Maybe when you see coffee appearing more and more in your food diary as you cut back on Coke, you'll notice that "Coffee" actually means a cup of coffee with two creams and two heaping teaspoons of sugar, plus a pastry. You're becoming more mindful.

So this food diary option means not to change anything from the first two weeks, but to create a mechanism to enhance your mindfulness about your performance.

The third possibility is that your weight tracking over two weeks doesn't show anything much; the results are ambiguous. There was probably that much variation in your weight when you weren't doing anything about food intake.

The truth is that ambiguous results are pretty negative. At this point we're trying out changes with the idea that our weight will show some significant downward trend. If it doesn't, it's natural to feel disappointed. Read over the three options for Scenario 2 above, and decide which of them you want to apply to your situation.

My guess is that if you have been reading this book attentively and following each step from Chapter I on, you are solidly in Scenario 1. The reason I think so is that losing a little weight initially is pretty easy. People do it all the time. So don't let these initial steps upset your equanimity too much in either direction: euphoria or depression.

You're in the groove. Keep it up. At the end of each week, look over the results, think about your week in the context of your overall goals for the three month period, and decide where you want to be at the end of next week and how you plan to get there.

Here's your take-away for this chapter:

Fast weight loss is the kiss of death. Slow, incremental, consistent loss is the key to long term success in weight management. Losing three pounds in three months can be much harder than losing three pounds in three weeks.

Chapter IX. Mindfulness and Daily Life

Sometimes people who are attracted to meditation think that meditation begins and ends on the meditation mat. You meditate half an hour once or twice a day, and you wait for wisdom and peacefulness to take over your life.

Meditation may well have clear, direct, and early effects on your life; if you meditate regularly it inevitably will over time. But most programs or teachers of mindfulness meditation include other areas of your life as essential and explicit, not accidental or incidental, parts of the "practice" of meditation. There are three main areas of life affected by a mindfulness practice: ethical practice; development of a focused, calm, and clear mind; and the development of insight or wisdom. These three aspects of mindfulness necessarily work together.

It's not very practical to expect your sitting meditation to give you a focused, calm, and clear mind if you are more or less deliberately engaging in practices you yourself consider unethical. Nor is it likely that you can achieve major insights about yourself without a certain amount of mental clarity and focus. The process of developing a meditation practice typically resembles a spiral that twines these three aspects together.

Hopefully as you read the preceding paragraphs you were thinking: "Hey, didn't we already cover this?" Good for you! You're remembering that way back in Chapter III I talked about moving back and forth between focus or concentration of mind on the one hand and insight on the other hand. And then in Chapter V there was the long discussion about the Eightfold Path and the Five Rules of Life.

Now that you have entered The Groove in terms of your food management practices, it's time to revisit the integration of your meditation practice with the rest of your life, including your food management practice. Throughout this book, and potentially for the rest of your life, you'll be reminded that there's really only one practice, and it involves balancing all aspects of your life.

The one thing I recommend you try based on this chapter is to consciously move mindfulness off your meditation cushion and into your daily life. No need to make a big deal of this. It's just a matter of pulling your attention from whatever you're doing and to take a minute to focus on your breathing and on your exact current state of being and doing. I'll give you a couple of examples.

What do you do and how do you feel when you're driving and you are stopped at a red light? What if you started using red lights like the little mindfulness bells you'll hear in some meditation retreats or sessions? Try this or something similar. Establish a link between something in your daily life and your mindfulness practice. Then when you find yourself at a red light, or whatever that daily life trigger is for you, call your attention to your breathing for a few breaths. As you breathe and notice your breathing, you can do a quick body and mind scan. How is your body feeling right now? What's going on with your thoughts and feelings?

Or pick some routine activity in your day and just pay attention to it. I find making a bed a perfect activity for this. Washing dishes is excellent as well. I've heard some people use brushing their teeth. The idea is to do whatever it is with total immediate attention to what you're doing. So what's different about that, you may ask. Don't you always pay attention to what you're doing? Check this out for yourself. What is your brain doing while you brush your teeth? Or making the bed? Most of us find, when we do this, that our Monkey Mind is totally in charge, which normally means it is operating in either the past or the future. Some people refer to repetitious activities of this kind as "mindless activity." The way to take away that time from the Monkey Mind is to make it mindful. Try paying precise attention to exactly what you're doing. Straighten out that sheet and tuck it in mindfully. It's just a way to remind yourself to recover your present moments.

In my own search for balance in this book between its two focuses, meditation and weight management, I find it necessary to keep reminding you, my ideal reader, that meditation is primary, weight management secondary. Meditation is the means; weight management is the end. This balance between the two doesn't just represent a personal preference on my part. It reflects the way the world works: meaningful change starts on the inside and is reflected externally. That's why so many people get such unsatisfactory results from so many diets.

It's not even exactly right to say that weight management is the end, because meditation isn't as goal-oriented as that would imply. There's a paradox at the heart of meditation that I finally have to own up to. Maybe by this point you've already encountered it in your own practice.

Meditation is a form of not-doing. In its essence, it involves turning loose of results, releasing the future, living in the present. Going into meditation with the attitude that you are going to define its outcomes in your life is just another way of turning your future over to your Monkey Mind. If your Monkey Mind was capable of moving you toward balance in your life, why aren't you there already? Who do you think has been in charge up to now?

Beginning to meditate is always to a large extent an act of faith. The difference between this particular act of faith and the leap of faith associated with religious practices is that the object of the faith is not outside yourself. Nor is it absolute. It is provisional, experimental, experiential. Mediation in the Vipassana tradition doesn't involve believing in the absolute truth of what the Buddha taught. It involves trying something out. Vipassana invites you to try out a practice. It says: "This is the way we think the world works. Try it out; see for yourself. We think that managing your life in a certain way leads to positive results. Try it out; see for yourself. We don't think the Monkey Mind is a very good guide to happiness. Here are some ways that have been effective for some people to find alternatives to the Monkey Mind. Try them out; see for yourself."

The driving idea in this book is that there is a subtle but powerful and eminently practical effectiveness in this practice. Vipassana meditation is a perfect antidote to the prevalent unhealthy aspects of Western civilization and its discontents: violence; unhealthy dependence on alcohol and/or on legal and illegal drugs; extreme consumerism; unsatisfactory personal relationships; increase in chronic mental and physical health problems. But don't take my word for it. Try it out; see for yourself.

The personal discovery I want to share with you is that this simple practice supports health in direct and surprising ways. If your weight is symptomatic of imperfect health, a meditation practice will support your practical attempts to do something about it. If there are obstacles in your body or in your mind to healthful practices with regard to food and weight, meditation will help you understand and resolve them. This is equally true with regard to other issues: personal relationships; financial management; professional and career issues.

Let me repeat for emphasis: **a meditation practice will support your practical attempts to manage any aspect of your life in a healthy direction.** It's not magical. You still have to take the practical steps that promote health. In the area of weight management, you still have to create a framework as described in previous chapters and methodically follow the steps involved in a longterm weight management program. Your meditation practice will support you. Try it out; see for yourself.

If meditation involves releasing the future and giving up the idea of defining results in advance, how can it be expected to create specific positive results in our life? That's the paradox, a paradox that has also been found to be operative in the practice of Western psychology. Being able to make personal changes requires self-acceptance just as you are. Total acceptance of your present makes it possible to change your future.

As you follow the directions in this book related to weight management, you are recording and paying attention to immediate measurable results. Effect follows cause clearly and simply. Is the same thing true in your meditation practice? Far from it! In fact, the on-the-pillow meditation is opposite in many ways to not only your weight management techniques but also to the ways we are taught to manage other aspects of Western life.

Take goal-setting, for example.

In the chapters on weight management, I have encouraged you to be specific and intentional, to set short-term goals and to pay attention every day to the relationship between your present reality and your goals.

In your meditation practice, this is neither possible nor desirable. The title of one of the books listed in Appendix 3 is "Being Nobody, Going Nowhere." Setting goals is about managing the past and the future, the "before" you and the "after" you. The immediate practice of sitting meditation is about present mindfulness, the "now" you.

When you sit in meditation, your focus is on the present. It is accepting; it is noticing without judgment. It is relaxing. It is not trying for something. It is not focused on being or wanting to be different in any way from exactly the way you are in this present moment.

Sitting still on a regular basis, mindful of precisely what is going on with you in the present, initiates a dynamic and profound process. Being mindful of and accepting of whatever is going on in the present, without judgment or striving, orients your mind and body in a space that automatically allows and facilitates a process of unfolding that our normal ways of operating in the world prevent or hinder.

The simple fact of regular sitting meditation is more important than the specific techniques of meditation you choose to practice. The particular book you read or meditation group you join may teach you to follow the breath going into and out of your nose; or to repeat a mantra; or to focus on a koan; or to focus on a candle flame or a particular object; or to note and label the thoughts that you observe passing through your mind. Any of these techniques may be useful to you. What is most important, however, is to sit still on a regular (daily) basis and to be mindful without judgment or striving or attachment to what is happening in the immediate present.

This relaxation of judgment is profoundly therapeutic. It gives permission to your entire organism with all its defined and indefinable aspects to move toward healthy balance. Your ego mind or Monkey Mind cannot do this, but there is present in you, perhaps concealed or confused by layers of accretions, a wisdom that has never left you and which will emerge if you create the space for its subtle voice and healing influence.

One could argue that a person who wants to access this healing process and who also has specific elements of his life in which he would like to experience that healing support should first establish a firm foundation in the meditation practice before trying to effect specific changes. Some readers may wish to do exactly that: to focus on establishing a sitting meditation practice for six months or a year before attempting a new approach to weight management.

Others may find that simultaneously applying mindfulness methods to a specific practice like weight management actually facilitates the sitting meditation practice by grounding it immediately in meaningful ways in daily life. Each person must make that judgment based on his or her individual experience.

The one caution I would emphasize is that if you try to simultaneously establish a meditation practice and experiment with the mindfulness method of weight management, don't give up on the method if your weight management goals prove initially to be beyond your abilities. If you experience more frustration than satisfaction during the first three months of your weight management program, step back from it and concentrate for three months or six months on the sitting meditation. Then try again.

I had been meditating for about a year before I decided to lose some weight. At the time, I didn't make any conscious connection between weight management and meditation until I noticed how different and how much easier managing my weight was now than it used to be. When I paid attention, the connection became clear. But I don't really know from personal experience whether it will work as well if you start meditation and weight management simultaneously. Try it out. See for yourself.

Here's your Chapter IX take-away:

Going into meditation with the attitude that you are going to define its outcomes in your life is just another way of turning the future over to your Monkey Mind. Meditation doesn't operate based on defined future outcomes. It unfolds based on its own powerful, subtle, and non-linear dynamic.

Chapter X. Maintaining Your Target Weight

In this chapter we take up two issues that were brought up and deferred earlier in the book: how to identify and maintain your target or ideal weight; and the role exercise plays in losing weight and maintaining your ideal weight.

What is your ideal weight? How do you decide what it is? We deferred that issue in Chapter IV, primarily because making that determination requires a higher level of mindfulness than one would normally have at the beginning of a mindfulness meditation practice. But at some point, as you get closer to your ideal weight, you'll have to decide when enough is enough.

I recommend that you take into consideration a combination of factors. First and most important, if you have used the mindfulness method to get your weight into the neighborhood of the ideal, use your mindfulness to pinpoint your final goal. How do you feel at your current weight? How do you look to yourself? How do you feel about other people's opinions of your weight and looks? When you meditate and focus on your body, what's your verdict?

Second, if you have a regular doctor, what is her advice? Many physicians recommend to their patients that they lose weight in the interest of various health issues. (In my experience, they are at least mildly shocked if you actually do lose weight as directed.) Your doctor may be a helpful advisor, especially if you have inclinations toward excessive weight loss. It's quite possible to get so excited to find you can actually decide what you will weigh that you literally don't know when to quit. With our society putting before us models of beauty, especially feminine beauty, tending toward the anorexic, a professional opinion about your ideal healthy weight can be a valuable corrective.

Finally, perhaps the most common current guide for healthy weight is something called the body mass index. Charts based on this computation are less than totally dependable because they are based on only height and weight, not body type, and the weight categories of "normal," "overweight," "obese," and "extremely obese" are in some cases too broad to be very useful.

For example, a chart I'm looking at now says that if you are 64 inches tall (5'4"), you are "overweight" if you weigh between 145 and 169 pounds. That's somewhat useful, but how about the "normal" range from 110 to 144 pounds? For my own height of 72" the "normal" range is from 140 to 183. I know from experience that 140 pounds looks and feels way too thin, and if I were looking to this chart for guidance about my ideal weight, the range of 43 pounds within "normal" wouldn't be very helpful.

As a societal index, the body mass index chart is at least helpful to indicate for each height (in inches) the lowest weight that is considered overweight. Here's an extract of that information:

Height	Overweight
58	119
59	124

60	128
61	132
62	136
63	141
64	145
65	150
66	155
67	159
68	164
69	169
70	174
71	179
72	184
73	189
74	194
75	200
76	205

If you're interested in getting more information about this index, Google "Body Mass Index".

When you're in the process of losing weight, especially if you started out thirty or more pounds overweight, you just work at staying in the groove as described in Chapters VI and VIII, and watch your weight settling down, pound by pound. The least of your worries is exactly where to stop, or how to maintain your weight at the ideal level once you get there. Once you do figure out what your target weight is and eventually arrive there, you might feel that you're done: your problems are over and you can relax. It might surprise you to find out that, at least for some people, maintaining weight at the ideal level is quite different from losing weight, and initially can even be more difficult.

The length of time it takes you to reach the weight you have identified as your ideal weight may be important to you emotionally, but in the context of life-long mindfulness and weight management, it's relatively unimportant whether it takes you one year or five years. As long as you are on a path that moves you gradually and healthily toward your ideal weight, the process can be as enjoyable and rewarding as reaching your goal.

As I've mentioned a number of times, especially if you started out with a lot of excess weight, the most important factor in sustainable weight loss is to be slow and methodical. That way your mindfulness meditation has time to ensure that your entire organism can assimilate the weight loss as it happens by dealing with the emotional, psychological, and spiritual components that drove your body into overweight status in the first place. Your "habit energy" that resulted in too much weight is gradually offset and overcome by the special energy born of mindfulness.

Now let's get a little bit technical again. We'll need EP for this.

EP started out at 162 pounds, you remember, and her doctor had advised her that 162 was about 30 pounds too many. No need to go through all the vicissitudes of her process. By the time you get to your ideal weight, you could write your own book about it (I hope you will; I'd love to read it.). As EP approached the 30 pound loss after twenty months of mindfulness meditation and weight management, she decided her doctor had been about right. She rounded her target weight of 132 down to 130, and you can imagine her feelings when she saw the number 130 on her bathroom scale for the first time. She had been getting lots of comments from her friends about how terrific she looked, and she had to agree. She looked great!

And she felt better than she had felt in a long, long time. The main downside was the money she had spent replacing her wardrobe, but how painful could it really be to buy reduced size clothes to fit a reduced size body?

By the time you get to your target weight, you'll be pretty good at knowing what it takes to steadily lose weight. Knowing what it takes to maintain your weight is a little different. You're no longer making decisions about what and how much to eat in order to consume fewer calories than your body needs to sustain its current weight, but how to calibrate your intake of calories for maintenance. Once again, being specific with regard to your intentionality is key.

Let's say your target weight, like EP's, was 130 pounds. Last week for the first time in nine years, you saw that number on your scale. Now, what does it mean to maintain your weight at 130 pounds. I gave you a report on my own difficulties with this issue in Chapter VI. Remember, how you define maintaining your target weight is very important.

My own compromise solution was to say that I was committed to seeing my target number of 175 on my scale at least one time each week. That worked pretty well for me. It didn't give my monkey mind enough room to get too tricky. If I see the numbers drift (or jerk) upward, I know pretty much what I need to do.

A couple of years ago I changed my target weight to between 165 and 170. Last week I saw 168 four times, 167 twice and 166 once, so I know I'm doing OK. If you set your intention clearly and explicitly, you don't have to guess about how you're doing.

The important thing is to continue to be mindful, continue your meditation practice, continue to weigh and record your weight every day, pay attention to the results, pay attention to how you feel about it, and strategize as necessary to keep the positive results.

Be as experimental about maintaining your weight as you were about losing weight. EP started out feeling pretty sure that as long as she kept weighing herself every day, she would know if she started some negative trend with her weight management, and would be able to take action to correct it. So she didn't really define any precise rules about weight; just the general intention to maintain her weight at 130 pounds.

That worked fine for several months, but then she started noticing a pattern she didn't like. She would give herself permission to eat larger than usual dinners when special circumstances like parties or out-of-town visitors happened. Holidays especially would result in missed work-out sessions in addition to larger than usual meals. EP would respond to these "special" circumstances and the resultant larger numbers showing up on her scale by returning to her weight loss methods, but she wasn't happy that she had essentially returned to yo-yo dieting on a smaller scale. She couldn't help but notice that there were two or three week periods when all the numbers on her calendar were higher than 130.

She asked herself, "Why can't I enjoy myself during special situations without pigging out?" She noticed that she didn't even enjoy over-eating; in fact, it didn't really feel good or make her happy in any way. Luckily EP had maintained an excellent regular meditation practice. She was able to catch onto the fact that what was driving the overeating was pure "habit energy," specifically the identification of celebration with more and richer food.

She remembered the discussion in this book about specificity of intention, and went back and re-read the chapters where that is discussed. She decided to try the method I described for myself. She would ensure that no week passed without the number 130 showing up on her weight record at least once. She found that her mindfulness was sharper with that anchoring definition, and that the narrower focus on each single week helped her be more thoughtful about her eating patterns.

You'll need to go through your own process to make the switch from losing weight to maintaining weight when the time comes. Just don't be surprised if it requires some specific mindful attention.

Now let's pick up something important that I mentioned in Chapter IV and said I would discuss later.

I noted that there are two main choices for people who want to lose weight: to consume fewer calories or to burn more calories. I said that burning more calories is a fine thing, but suggested that you not concern yourself too much about burning more calories as a primary strategy for losing weight. Now, as promised, I'll explain why I take that approach.

When I walk my normal evening route of 3 ½ miles, it takes me about an hour. Hauling my 165 to 170 pounds 3 ½ miles in an hour burns about 350 calories. Ten walks burn about 3500 calories, or the equivalent of about one pound. If I do that walk on the average 2 ½ times per week, which is pretty close to what I do, I'm burning an extra 100 calories per day on the average. Do you know what the food equivalent of 100 calories is? Just over half a can of coke. Ten potato chips. Twenty corn chips. About 1/3 of a piece of pie.

Does exercising stimulate your appetite? You see the problem. Unless you are able to increase your exercise without a compensatory increase in calorie consumption, perhaps in the guise of a "reward" for good behavior, the balance of burning and consuming is not positive.

My mother-in-law, who was diabetic, took insulin daily for quite a few years. When we served a particularly tempting desert, she would say: "I'll have some of that. I'll just up the insulin a little tonight."

There's nothing easier than storing up credits for future exercise when you're tempted by a particularly tempting piece of bait: "I'll be OK. I'll just swim 30 extra laps this afternoon."

Regular exercise is absolutely necessary for your physical and mental well-being. But it's not a winner as your primary strategy for weight loss. That's why I've encouraged you not to concentrate on exercise for weight loss. It's just one more thing for your monkey mind to play games with. Concentrate on exercise for total fitness and health instead, and focus on calorie intake as your primary strategy for weight loss. Any extra loss or additional fitness and improved appearance from regular exercising is a bonus.

Once you're at your target or ideal weight, you're in a better position to integrate your calorie control and your exercise regimen.

For one thing, you've demonstrated conclusively that you are in control of how much you weigh. You've learned some important, more general, things in your meditation about how you operate. You can focus your mindfulness more skillfully. You can broaden your focus and pay more attention not only to weight, but to fitness and general health. You can focus less exclusively on weight, and pay more attention to shape and tone.

None of this is as "all or nothing" as I've described it here. Most of us, as we demonstrate some success in losing unwanted pounds, are already paying more attention to the quality of what we eat and how much exercise we get. It's just a matter of priorities. Given our limited ability to pay attention, it makes sense initially to concentrate on weight. General fitness and health will take on their rightful importance in our lives once we've succeeded in taming weight.

Exactly how did you go about losing that first pound? There will be as many answers as there are readers. That's as it should be; you are the creator of your own body, on a daily basis. How do you achieve fitness? That's not what this book is about, but I would expect the answers would vary as much as the answers about losing that first pound.

My wife loves swimming. If I'm going to get wet, I want it to be in the controlled environment of my shower. When I go to the beach near our house, what I appreciate about it isn't that there's a big ocean to jump into, but the fact that the beach extends an uninterrupted four miles or more, a wonderful place to walk.

I've always liked hard physical labor, and I don't care if it's hot. My wife can't tolerate much sun, and some of my projects look like a mild form of insanity to her. She likes to get up early and go to a yoga or exercise class. I think jumping into activity first thing in the morning is highly unnatural.

The point is that it doesn't matter. It's important to get regular and adequate exercise. It's not so important what form it takes.

One more thing. As you think about maintaining your target weight, you might want to go back to Chapter VI and re-read the part about food quality. Like exercise, improving the quality of your food intake is something that mindfulness will lead you to more or less automatically. The discussion in Chapter VI is a minimalist version. I encourage you to look in the bibliography at the end of the book for a listing of a few books that take up the issue of food quality from a number of different directions. Mindfulness is more effective if it's informed by expert information.

Mindful Message: You are the creator of your own body on a daily basis.

Chapter XI. Change and Self-Esteem

Personal change, like organizational change, is a tricky business, and requires some strategy and some management. That's because, as we've already discussed briefly, organisms are what they are for good reasons. They have come to a certain equilibrium for an adequate set of causes or reasons, and it's not always easy to understand the reasons that underlay the current reality.

In terms of weight management, as we discussed in Chapter IV, there is a set of physical, psychological, and spiritual factors that have determined that your current weight is the "right" weight for you. You may not agree with the decision your whole organism has made that this is the right weight for you, and you may not understand many or most of the factors that created that decision. That's why you need some process like mindfulness meditation to help you slowly unwind the tangle of factors that determine your weight; to help you begin, slowly but surely, to weaken and undermine and eliminate some of the factors that have driven your weight in the past.

One of the fascinating pieces of this process, a piece that is in some ways central to the process, is the complicated constellation of factors commonly referred to as "self-esteem." How do we see ourselves? What do we think of ourselves? How do we feel about who we are and what we do? Are there things about ourselves that we "hate" or are "disgusted" by or reject as parts of ourselves? Are there things about ourselves that we take great pride in and treasure as our prime virtues or the characteristics that we see as intrinsic to our self-worth?

Have you ever said or heard someone else say "I hate it when I do that"? Or "I hate my body." Or "I hate my weight." Or "I hate my lack of discipline." What does it really mean to separate out some part or aspect of yourself to disown or to disrespect? And if you hate something about yourself, why is it so hard to change that particular something?

We've hinted in this book at the answers to some of these questions, each of which might deserve its own book, but we have said from the beginning that we were going to take you back to the basics. This chapter is attempting to take you back to the basics of change and self-esteem.

If you don't already have good or high self-esteem, why is that, and what would be necessary to change it?

Let's say your story to yourself about why you don't have good self-esteem goes something like this:

"I'm forty-two years old, 5 feet 6 inches tall, and weigh 185. I've been overweight since I was a teenager, and I've been called fat by other people and myself that whole time. I've tried everything I could think of to get my weight under control, but nothing has worked. Every time I see myself in the mirror, I can't see anything but all those extra pounds. To me they stand for all the things I dislike: being unhealthy; lacking discipline; being lonely; being physically unattractive; being out of control. How could I feel good about myself when that's what I see?"

If I asked you, "What are some things about yourself that you like," what would you say? I'll put some words in your mouth, but you should come up with your own answer. You might say: "There are actually quite a few things I like about myself. I think I'm a really good friend to my friends. I'm a good listener and a good communicator. I'm plenty smart and I'm well-educated. I have a Master's degree in Communications, and I have a great career going in that field. I'm a good and valued employee. My parents are both still alive and I have close relationships with both of them. But the truth is that I see all my good characteristics as somehow separate from myself, but I **feel** my negative characteristics, especially my weight, as who I really am every day."

The sad truth is that one or two failings that are highly emotionally laden can provide a generally negative coloring to a composite self-image that has lots of positives about it. But let's look a little more closely into how that works.

When you list the things about yourself that you feel good about, everything you mention—being a good friend, good employee, smart, loyal, good daughter—is truly and even universally "esteem-able," or, to use Webster's preferred version, estimable.

Likewise, when you list the things that make you feel bad about yourself—overweight, out of control, physically unattractive (at least in comparison to

112

how you would look at your ideal weight), undisciplined, lonely, unhealthy—these are characteristics that wouldn't be on anybody's list of things they are striving for. They are not generally considered estimable.

Now here's the core of the issue. **People, including those who should know better, like to try to tell you that you shouldn't feel that way.** Look at the good things, they tell you. Focus on the positive. Don't dwell on things you can't change. Don't feel bad about yourself. Work on your self-esteem.

But you know as long as it's you, looking through your eyes and feeling your feelings, you will not look at yourself in the mirror and feel good about what you see. **To you, what you see is not estimable.** Other people may look at you and like you or love you and see only your sterling qualities. When you look at yourself, in your deepest feelings, you are sadly lacking in some qualities that are very important to you.

I'm hammering away at this, maybe excessively, because I think this view of self-esteem is so important, and is so misunderstood and misrepresented in self-help literature and in the popular sociology and psychology of our society.

Self-esteem is not a separate issue from what is truly estimable and how you truly see yourself. People typically have low self-esteem because they see things about themselves that are truly not estimable, things they have struggled unsuccessfully to change.

If I didn't believe deeply that personal change, even change at very deep and basic levels of the self, is possible, I would have to admit that my view of self-esteem is pretty depressing. But since I'm quite sure that **personal change, and specifically change for you involving management of your weight, is within your power,** I think there are enormous grounds for optimism.

What's not possible, in my view, is to lie to yourself about the dhamma, about what is, about how reality really works, and on the basis of that delusion to effect meaningful positive change. Understanding how your world works makes changing how it works feasible for you.

That's the whole point of insight or mindfulness meditation. The only subject and the only object of your meditation is your personal reality. It's purely about what feels unsatisfactory about your life; about the cause of the unsatisfactory aspects of your life; about the way out, for you personally, of the unsatisfactory aspects of your life; and about the specific path that puts you as a unique individual on the way to happiness.

Do you recognize in that last paragraph the Four Noble Truths of the Buddha? They are usually abbreviated (apparently first by the Buddha himself) as Dissatisfaction; Cause; End; Path. Less compactly, the Truths are that human life is characterized by unsatisfactoriness; that there is a cause for that (attachment); that it's possible to end that unsatisfactoriness by dealing accurately with its cause; and that there is a path from unsatisfactoriness to happiness. The fourth Noble Truth refers to the Eightfold Path to Happiness which I've already talked about in several chapters.

Your dhamma, your truthful reality, is that you weigh more than you want to weigh and it makes you unhappy and it makes you feel bad about yourself.

People commonly talk about estimable personal characteristics as if they were innate, permanent, inexplicable aspects of character. "You're so disciplined," they will say, as if the actions they are observing are the automatic and effortless results of something **you** were given and **they** were deprived of. "You're lucky. You don't have weight problems," a friend told me, as if "trimness" was some god-given quality that required no involvement on my part. Worse, the implication was that she had not, for reasons beyond her control, been infused with that quality.

So let's say that you suffer from "low self-esteem," and the quality you most identify in yourself as responsible is "lack of discipline." What that usually means is that there are things you would like to do, or at least that you would like to have done, but you never actually get up the energy or motivation to do that thing. "I would like to; I just don't have the discipline," you tell your friends.

Let's put some content on this. Let's say that you dropped out of college after your Freshman year because of a great employment opportunity. The opportunity didn't work out as you had imagined, and since then you've worked in jobs that don't really challenge you or satisfy you. You've always regretted not finishing college, and you've talked about going back to school, but somehow it never quite seemed possible. You'd like to continue your education, but you just don't have the discipline to do it. And your opinion of yourself, your self-esteem, seems to center around this failure.

Once you identify something as a source of poor self-esteem, what can you do about it? Typically, whatever it is, lack of education or being overweight or lack of financial success, looms very large or heavy in your consciousness of it. You might feel doomed to stay uneducated, overweight, or poor, and it might feel that the root of that condition is lack of discipline.

My working hypothesis is that even more basic and foundational to character than being uneducated, overweight, or poor, even more basic than lack of discipline, is a failure of mindfulness. That's why other people, often with growing exasperation, keep telling you: "There's no reason for you to feel that way. All you need to do is X, Y, and Z, and your problem would be solved." Your problems, to your friends, are not unique or particularly intractable. They're not even very complicated.

Unsatisfactoriness comes to human beings in an infinite variety of forms. That's why Freud could contrast the common ordinary misery of humans to real, clinical depression. Your own individual unsatisfactoriness is unique to you, and so is the path out of it.

If one of the manifestations in your life of unsatisfactoriness is being overweight, your "overweightness" is also unique to you. To think you could change a basic quality of unsatisfactoriness in your life without understanding to some extent the complex and multi-faceted causes of it is not realistic. Ending the specific quality of unsatisfactoriness without ending some of the causes of that quality defies the basic cause and effect relationship. And the Path onto which you must place your foot is also your own unique Path, which no one else can find and walk for you.

The beauty of the process is that you don't need to see very far ahead of yourself. You only need to be able to see far enough ahead to take the next step. Insight meditation does not provide illumination of the whole path; actually, that might be no more than a distraction from the next step.

Let's step back, now, and understand as clearly as possible what this process has to do with self esteem. We'll focus on our basic topic: management of weight. Just keep in mind that this change process can apply equally to the other issues we used as examples: lack of education; poverty; lack of discipline.

At the beginning of Chapters I and II, I gave you very precise and simple instructions about what to do and exactly how to do it. I made myself obnoxious by insisting on the importance of following those instructions without variation. That's because your path forward was almost entirely un-illuminated by your own mindfulness. Still, you were able to put your feet on a path and take a few steps.

By the time you got to Chapter VI, the guidance was more general, and the specifics you required had to be provided by you. You had to identify your own unique food habits or patterns; you had to decide what would be a good pattern to change initially; you had to observe your own reactions, pay attention mindfully to both your scale and your own organism. Why could you do that? Because your own mindfulness meditation practice was beginning to provide at least weak glimmers of illumination.

When you first noticed that you had completed the two week preparation period before your weight management program formally started, how did that feel? Did you find your actions estimable? You may not have thought it was a big deal, but on some level, you registered that you had succeeded. You had for two weeks acted as if you were disciplined and were able to take the first important steps on a new path.

When you completed the first two weeks of your actual weight management program, or the first month, and you succeeded in achieving your first weight goals, how did you feel? If you felt good, that's because what you had done was estimable. Some tentative shaky increase in self-esteem had happened, though you may not have thought about it like that.

Our self-esteem automatically increases when we mindfully observe ourselves doing estimable things. When we temporarily fail or slide backward, our self-esteem takes a hit. We can't fool ourselves. We know that what we have just done was not estimable. Somebody else telling us

"That's OK. You're doing fine" is meaningless to us. We know when we have done something estimable and when we have failed.

Setting reasonable, even easy goals initially is important for precisely that reason. Succeeding is not just losing a pound; succeeding in losing a pound in the allotted period of time creates an incremental, essential message to ourselves. Strengthened by our mindfulness meditation practice, we are making meaningful change. That change feeds us and encourages us to continue on the path.

Mindfulness meditation empowers us to make targeted positive change. Positive change, mindfully observed, empowers us to continue the meditation practice. The illumination becomes more powerful; the next step begins to seem more inevitable. You're in the groove.

This is how lasting positive change happens. At some point it's like quitting smoking. Going back is unimaginable.

There are two basic teachings in Buddhist philosophy or psychology that I want to leave you with that are supportive of change and self-esteem. The first is rooted in concepts of the conscious mind and the unconscious mind that far pre-date Freudian psychology. The second relates to one of the four most important Buddhist virtues, variously translated as Loving Kindness or Loving Friendliness. (The other three are compassion, shared joy, and equanimity.)

Whatever happens in your conscious mind first happens in and then arises from your unconscious mind. It's like having tons of data in your computer's random access memory, and small working files that you are currently working with that you have accessed and are actively using.

When something happens to make you consciously feel compassionate, it's because the seeds of compassion in your unconscious have been accessed and are being actively and consciously engaged. Someone else, whose seeds of compassion are stunted or withered from lack of use, might see the same homeless person or crying child and feel hostility or annoyance.

When you feel angry, it's because something has aroused the seeds of anger in your unconscious. The seeds of anger, which you always carry with you, are suddenly accessed and made conscious. You say: "That really makes me angry," but all that has happened is that feelings you always harbor have suddenly been activated. Someone else may not become angry at all with the same stimulus; it just doesn't push their "Anger Button."

All the human feelings are present in all of us. We all have the seeds of patience and impatience; loving friendliness and hatred or anger; equanimity and imbalance; compassion and resentment; joy and sadness; generosity and stinginess; happiness and depression; sloth and industriousness; anxiety and calmness; and on and on.

Some of these seeds are more readily accessible to us than others. And why is that? Because they are better nourished and more frequently exercised. Do you know someone who always seems capable of reacting to situations with a positive and well-directed energy? Do you know someone whose dominant and habitual emotional energy is based on resentment or hostility? Do you know someone who is never rattled, whose emotional home base is in equanimity? Or the opposite, someone who quickly slides into hysterical over-reaction?

How about you? What seeds are most readily accessible to you?

These personal characteristics and leanings are not accidents. Cause and effect are at work here.

Nor is your current constellation of "seeds" permanent or unchangeable. If your compassion "seed" is plump and well-nourished, that's because you have valued it and exercised it and have made it a familiar friend. If you have a small, withered seed of equanimity, that's because that quality has not been valued, recognized, and nourished adequately in you. You can't access it readily because you haven't often accessed and used it in the past. Instead, you have perhaps nourished a kind of emotional volatility, a seeking of emotional extremes.

Just as we can exercise and develop our triceps, we can choose to nourish and develop the seeds of the qualities we value, and we can diminish and starve the seeds of qualities we would like to see diminish in ourselves.

As you may have noticed from the long list of qualities above, each quality has its opposite or off-setting quality. If you feel that greed or grasping or clutching at things is something you would like to weaken, the most effective approach is not to directly attack those qualities, but to nourish and strengthen their opposites. If you want to weaken greed, deliberately practice generosity. If you want to weaken resentment, work on appreciation and compassion.

In each aspect of your life, it is possible to identify through meditation and general mindfulness the specific qualities that you value and want to build and the opposite qualities you would like to diminish. Mindfulness increasingly will allow you to be aware early in the process when resentment or greed is triggered. Merely being aware that the seed of resentment has been stirred up in your unconscious mind and has surfaced into your consciousness is a first crucial step. Just noticing "Oh, there's my old friend resentment waking up" puts you in a position to oppose it with understanding or appreciation, or even just to notice and observe it with mindfulness.

Noticing impulsiveness as an issue with food can lead you to identifying its offsetting quality of thoughtfulness or deliberation. You're using mindfulness to weaken one of the qualities that perhaps contributed to your being overweight, and to strengthen a quality that will help your whole organism make a different decision about what your "right" weight is.

What seeds do you want to water today? What seeds do you notice stirring this morning? Do you sometimes wake up in the morning already in the middle of some dominant feeling or theme? Can you use your meditation to give that feeling some attention, not to fight it or deny it, but simply to give it your full mindful attention and see what it is?

My last piece of guidance for you in the realm of mindfulness mediation is really just one particularly important example of selective watering of the seeds in the unconscious.

The Bible identifies three primary virtues: faith, hope, and charity or love. And, the Bible says, "The greatest of these is charity." Buddhist philosophy or psychology is in full agreement. In Pali, the language of many of the writings about mindfulness meditation and Buddhist teachings, the word is "metta," translated as love, or loving kindness, or loving friendliness.

Some practitioners recommend that you begin every meditation with a centering prayer for metta, which goes like this:

"May I be well, happy, and peaceful. May no harm come to me. May no problems come to me. May no difficulties come to me. May I be successful in everything I do today. And may I have the patience, understanding, courage and determination to meet and overcome the inevitable problems, difficulties and failures of life that come to me today."

If you like, you can then direct this prayer to particular individuals in your life, or to all living creatures everywhere.

"May So and So be well, happy, and peaceful. May no harm come to her." Etc.

You can include people who are particularly problematic or difficult to deal with.

You may notice a major difference between this prayer and prayers in other religious traditions. There is no invocation of a higher being, no asking that anyone do anything for you or someone else. Rather, the focus is on intentionality. The Metta Prayer is a way of setting our intention.

If you have, with full mindfulness, tried to align yourself with the dhamma, the way things are, things you may be inclined to do during the day that might undermine your wellness, happiness, and peace, that might actually bring you harm, may create a dissonance with the Metta Prayer. The more strongly the Metta Prayer pervades your intention, the more likely you are to notice when resentment, anger, or greed puts you on a path incompatible with the prayer.

Similarly, if you have mindfully invoked Metta for somebody in your life, acting toward that person in a way that contradicts your prayer for them also creates that dissonance. As you become more mindful, the dissonance between "May no harm come to her" and the temptation to make some negative comment about her will give you pause.

There's no magic in this. It's just a way to remind yourself as you start your day that you are once more putting your foot on the Eightfold Path, and the more aligned you are with the dhamma of your own life, the more peaceful and happy and healthy you will be.

Mindful Message: May you be well, happy, and peaceful. May no harm come to you. May you be successful in everything you do.

Chapter XII. Balance

While there is no measure of progress in meditation as precise as a bathroom scale, there is a subtle metric. Equanimity, or balance, is a natural result of a life characterized by mindfulness.

The opposite of equanimity is struggle, often characterized by aversion. Aversion, you may remember, is the other side of the coin called attachment or desire, which Buddhist psychology considers the primary cause of suffering.

Equanimity and its opposite manifest themselves in all aspects of life. In a life characterized by increasing mindfulness, an individual will notice a gradual shift toward balance or equanimity, with a concomitant decrease in aversion or struggle. At the end of this chapter you will find more detail about exactly how this shift might specifically affect your weight management. But first, a little background about how it typically plays out in more general life issues.

One of the primary weapons against struggle, aversion, and desire is acceptance or surrender. That's one reason meditation, which focuses on the present rather than the past or future, is an effective counter to suffering. An individual whose life is out of balance is likely to relate to the past with regrets, blame, and guilt, and to the future with elements of desire, aversion, and fear.

When you sit in meditation and when you extend mindfulness to all aspects of your life, you gradually learn to live more fully in the present, and your attitude to the present is more likely to be characterized by acceptance or surrender. This dialectic plays itself out in a slow, mostly imperceptible way over relatively long periods of time.

Acceptance or surrender is not to be confused with complacency or passivity; it is positive and characterized by action and energy. Acceptance of the present reality is a pre-condition for balanced and effective action. Ideally, one's life would flow with little conscious effort; decisions would be made without agonizing or intellectual dithering. The flow is a natural result of mindfulness, because a person who is habitually mindful is in touch with her inner reality and accurately aware of external reality. Under those conditions, choices and decisions appear to almost make themselves. That's what being "in the flow" means.

Perhaps you know someone who seems to have an innate sense of the right thing to do in unexpected circumstances. She doesn't have an excessive respect for "correctness" or the opinion of authorities. Rather she has her own inner compass, a reliable personal wisdom about what is right or wrong, appropriate or out of place. Maybe you are such a person. This apparently effortless equanimity or balance is both the result and the evidence of mindfulness.

Not only is the process of attaining balance or equanimity normally pretty slow, it's not easy to keep track of where you are. That's primarily because in the nature of mindfulness meditation, the meditator is not able to define the goals or ends of mindfulness with any exactness. You'll remember that this is true because the planning or projecting function in human beings is dominated by the Ego or Monkey Mind.

Eastern philosophy and religion tend to focus on the path; Western philosophy and religion tend to focus on end states.

In mindfulness meditation and in weight management, the important thing is to put yourself onto the path and to maintain the journey. That's why the fourth of the Four Noble Truths is the Eightfold Path. It's the path that is the way out of suffering, not the end of the path or any generically defined end state that we need to pay a lot of attention to. Many meditation teachers believe it's a mistake to get hung up on the desire for Enlightenment, which is sometimes considered the end or goal of meditation. Getting attached to the concept of Enlightenment is not different from any other attachment or desire. It's just one more desire, one more source of suffering that pulls us away from mindfulness of the present.

When you place yourself on the path by beginning a meditation practice, you "practice" acceptance of the present, release of the past and future, surrender to the process. When you do that, your body and mind begin the process of unfolding, of releasing, of balancing. Sitting meditation causes things to begin to happen. If you place yourself on the path, you will not remain in the same place; inevitably you will begin to move, perhaps in fits and starts, perhaps imperceptibly most of the time, but forward on the path.

One thing that happens once you place yourself on the path is that elements of imbalance in your being will begin to reveal themselves. They will present themselves for resolution. You may experience physical resistance, which can be resolved through standard meditation techniques discussed in all the books on meditation. You will certainly encounter intellectual resistance, periods when your Monkey Mind works hard to convince you that to continue to meditate represents a form of insanity.

Many people are so intimidated by the obstacles they can already see in themselves, or by obstacles that represent various misunderstandings of the process of meditation, that they are at least temporarily unable even to place themselves on the path. Many people react to the idea of a meditation practice by saying something like: "Oh, I couldn't do that. My mind is too chaotic to ever be still." This is simply a recognition that they are human beings and their Monkey Minds are in charge. Human beings predictably feel that their minds are too chaotic ever to be still. Or they may feel that their lives are too busy to take even half an hour a day to "do nothing."

As in most forms of physiological and psychological therapy, sources of imbalance or pain emerge as part of the process. Physical and/or psychological health may require that those elements of the whole person be integrated in some constructive way. This is very likely to occur in mindfulness meditation as well, and the acceptance, surrender, and release facilitated by meditation are effective tools in dealing with whatever emerges.

We discussed briefly in Chapter IV the possible relationship between weight issues and deep psychological issues. Chapter IX and this chapter have added necessary groundwork for an additional important point about this relationship.

One reason I suggest simultaneously placing yourself on the path of mindfulness meditation and the path of successful weight management is that those paths can have significant overlap, and traveling one path may support the other. Here's how.

You may remember the discussion in Chapter IV about how failure to deal with the underlying personal issues related to weight are one reason people can lose weight but not maintain their weight at the desired level. Those issues exert a strong gravitational force that represents all the physical and psychological reasons you were over your ideal weight in the first place. When you lose some weight, that gravitational force persistently tries to pull you back toward the higher weight.

Being on the path of mindfulness meditation creates another source and form of energy. The gravitational force pulling you back toward your old weight represents an imbalance in your being. It represents obstacles, physical and/or psychological, to health and balance. It represents issues which, if not brought into balance, will continue to pull you back to the unhealthy weight you now recognize as a symptom of organic imbalance, an imbalance in your own organism.

The practice of meditation gives you a new tool with which to deal with that imbalance, whatever its roots. Whatever "comes up" as you begin to lose a few pounds can be recognized, accepted, paid attention to, released, and resolved just like anything else that pops up along the path.

This is another reason underlying the statement in Chapter IV that fast weight loss is the enemy. Mindfulness meditation, by its very nature and due to the depth at which it works, creates real change in a very gradual way, at a pace regulated by the entire organism that you are. Forcing change in one facet of your being faster than your entire organism can deal with it and balance it simply invites relapse.

Especially at the beginning of your mindfulness weight management process, it's important to give the meditation part of the process time to keep up. Spending the first three or six months simply stabilizing your weight, or perhaps reducing it slightly, allows you to practice and perfect the mechanical aspects of weight management and to make them routine. It also gives you time to get deeply enough into meditation to begin, slowly and subtly, to achieve enough equanimity or balance to deal with the issues that surface as you lose the first increments of weight.

That extra weight has perhaps been protecting you against something. As you begin to mindfully release that protection, your meditation practice helps to create a new balance in the organism, the person you are becoming, who no longer needs that protection. That's the anti-relapse dynamic that mindfulness meditation, along with weight management, provides.

One reason change can be so disturbing is that it disrupts whatever aspect of organic equilibrium it affects. Change, of necessity, happens in predictable stages: change; re-balancing; stasis. As you develop your meditation practice and stay in the groove of weight management, you will in fact experience these three stages over and over. The regulatory mechanisms of such a complex organism as a human being manage this in an almost miraculous way. In a normally healthy human being, those mechanisms will not permit imbalances of such severity that the overall mental and physical health is jeopardized.

The healthy norm is small change, rebalancing, stasis; additional incremental change, rebalancing, stasis. You may well be experiencing this repetitive pattern in many ways, some too subtle for you to perceive and understand. You can trust yourself. Unless you proceed in obviously abrupt, dislocating, or extreme ways, the complex organism that you are is very well equipped to manage your process. And if you are too extreme in some way, those very regulatory mechanisms will let you know in no uncertain terms that you need to slow down, moderate your approach, allow yourself to unfold at a healthy pace.

Your relationship to food may well participate in this change, rebalancing, stasis. Here are a few patterns that it might be worth your while to have some advance knowledge of.

How does imbalance, lack of equanimity, struggle, aversion manifest itself in weight management?

The primary manifestation, of course, is being overweight itself. Your own body has become an object of aversion and struggle. The imbalance is implicit in the very structure of your body. The body's natural tendency toward health is jeopardized in the hundred ways excess weight has been identified as a major risk factor in heart disease, diabetes, musculoskeletal problems, and many other health disorders.

Being overweight dramatizes on a stage visible to the whole world the imbalance and struggle between your conscious mind, your unconscious, and your body. The body, yielding to mostly unconscious promptings, seems to have a mind of its own, and your conscious desires to exert control over the body's actions are frustrated by factors of which you have limited awareness. It is not uncommon for this aversion and struggle to persist for an entire lifetime.

Being anorexic or bulimic are simply opposite sides of the coin, equal manifestations of imbalance and struggle.

Lack of equanimity sometimes shows itself in daily and weekly eating patterns, perhaps in cycles of binges and remorseful starvation, sometimes in extreme desire for and focus on certain types of foods, with aversions and disgust for others.

Cycles of despair over the failure of the last miracle diet and irrational hope in the next betray a lack of consistency and balance.

The way food issues can come to dominate one's mind and obtrude themselves into every conversation, wanted or not, attests to a failure of equanimity.

Extreme swings in food habits and practices may be a symptom of imbalance and struggle. This may be as simple as a practice of skipping breakfast or lunch for a couple of weeks, then a shift to making breakfast the main meal of the day. Swings between overeating and fasting are not only generally unhealthy, they betray unhealthy and unbalanced attitudes toward food and toward your body.

Today a vegetarian, tomorrow a vegan, the next day an omnivore. Either one or all of them may be excellent choices, but a frantic search for the perfect weight by searching for the perfect dietary framework simply shows that internal balance or equanimity is lacking.

It might be valuable for you to look thoughtfully at your life through this lens and to specifically identify imbalances and struggles you associate with weight management. Then, as your mindfulness practice deepens, you will find yourself being mindful of those imbalances **as they manifest themselves**. Your mindfulness can almost be measured in terms of the length of time between a manifestation of imbalance and awareness of that manifestation.

Thoughts and words arise first in the unconscious, then emerge in your conscious mind and perhaps in language. Let's say your imbalance and struggle with weight and food typically manifest themselves through frequent venting in conversations. If you were perfectly mindful, you would see this happen in the moment of emergence, and you would "have the presence of mind" to be able to decide whether to complete the act of speaking about food or not.

The gap in time between the manifestation of imbalance and your mindfulness of it is a measure of your degree of equanimity and mindfulness.

As the "mindfulness shift" begins to happen, you may find yourself saying: "Oh God, I just did it again. I've been on the phone with my friend for fifteen minutes, and I must have gone on about food and dieting for at least ten. Oh yeah, I did the same thing last night with Jerry." You are becoming more mindful. You have recognized in general that you talk a lot about food and dieting, and now you're starting to pick up on individual instances of that happening. Before long you may catch yourself in the act and say to your friends, "Enough about that. Let's talk about something else." Your recognition is getting closer to the actual happening.

At some point you will notice that you're about to bring up your weight in conversation, and you'll decide not to. You are practicing mindfulness of the mouth. You are taking a mindful step on the Eightfold Path.

This is the nature of the shift toward equanimity, by way of mindfulness. The changes you make will be powered not by "will power," to be reversed when your conscious attention flags. The changes will emerge in your life, powered by mindfulness, fueled by a consistent mindfulness meditation practice.

If you consciously identify patterns of imbalance and struggle in your weight management, and then begin to become more and more immediately aware of manifestations of those patterns, you are moving mindfulness from your meditation cushion into your life.

One word of caution. In meditation, when you become aware that your mind has wandered away from the object of meditation, you are taught to gently bring it back to the breath or other object. This should be done without mentally chastising yourself, blaming yourself for lack of concentration, etc. The same attitude applies to noticing that you have once more exhibited some evidence of imbalance or struggle. Getting emotionally down on yourself, beating yourself up, gives more power to the imbalance. Simply take note of what happened, "barely notice" it, and move on. Don't over-involve yourself in what has happened.

One more example of equanimity in weight management, and I'm through. I want to clarify the difference between equanimity and struggle by showing you how one and the same action can be the result of either, depending on your relationship to the action.

As an example of imbalance, I mentioned above a pattern of over-eating and then fasting. Fasting in this pattern is usually an act of hostility and punishment, hardly a positive action based on mindfulness.

Fasting, however, can be a powerful tool for mindfulness, if it is mindfully built into your patterns of weight management. For example, you might think of a day of fasting every two weeks or once a month as a regular part of your weight management plan. You might choose to fast on a day that you can devote to quiet and restful activities, perhaps with an extra period or two of meditation.

You might want to pay particular attention to how fasting affects your energy, your moods, your thoughts and feelings. You could combine a day of fasting with an expression of loving friendliness toward people for whom adequate food is a daily issue, perhaps by a gift to a Food Bank or an organization that serves the homeless.

Occasional fasting can be a wonderful experience of mindfulness, not an extreme or punitive reaction to past excesses.

You can experiment with various types of fasting. I recommend avoiding extreme fasts. Adequate fluids should always to permitted. Diets don't have to be absolute; they don't even have to involve hunger, which might sound contradictory. A form of diet I particularly find appealing simply eliminates "bait," forms of food that we eat not out of hunger but because their taste is particularly tempting. Here's an example:

Take a cup or so of wheat berries and soak them overnight before the day of your fast. In the morning cook them until they're plump and soft but still chewy. Make sure you have a good source of fruit, preferably not citrus. Fuji apples are perfect. Your day of fasting allows you to have all the water, wheat berries, and apples you want. Eat and drink mindfully.

Make up your own fasts. Maybe you'll want to call on a day of fasting sometime when your weight seems to be stuck on a particular number regardless of what you do. Just make sure the fast isn't followed by a day when you eat more than normal.

I'm hoping that as you, my ideal readers, come up with your own creative ways to manage your weight, you'll call up my blog and share your insights and discoveries. I can't think of any better result for this book than a sangha, a community of practitioners, sharing with me and each other your experiences with mindful weight management.

Mindful Message: The path of mindfulness meditation and the path of successful weight management have significant overlap. Mindfully traveling both paths simultaneously allows each path to support the other.

Appendix A. RECOMMENDED READING

I. Books on Mindfulness and Meditation. Each of the books in this section develops a different aspect of insight meditation. Many of them reward repeated readings.

Buddhadasa Bhikku. 1996. <u>Mindfulness with Breathing: A Manual for Serious Beginners</u>. Boston: Wisdom Publications. This is an excellent second introduction to meditation. It's quite different from <u>Mindfulness in Plain English</u>, somewhat more technical. It provides a great survey of the 16 step formal meditation structure of the Vipassana tradition.

Buddhadasa Bhikku. 1994. <u>Heartwood of the Bodhi Tree: The Buddha's Teaching on Voidness</u>. Boston: Wisdom Publications.

Clifford, Patricia Hart. 1994. <u>Sitting Still: An Encounter with Christian Zen.</u> Mahwah, New Jersey: Paulist Press.

Gunaratana, Henepola. 1994. <u>Mindfulness in Plain English</u>. Boston: Wisdom Publications.

Gunaratana, Henepola. 2001. <u>Eight Mindful Steps to Happiness.</u> Boston: Wisdom Publications.

Johnson, Will. 1996. <u>The Posture of Meditation: A Practical Manual for Meditators of All Traditions.</u> Boston: Shambhala.

Rosenberg, Larry. 2004. Breath by Breath: The Liberating Practice of Insight Meditation. Boston: Shambhala.

Thich Nhat Hanh. 1996. Breathe! You Are Alive: Sutra on the Full Awareness of Breathing. Berkeley: Parallax Press.

Thich Nhat Hanh. 2001. Anger: Wisdom for Cooling the Flames. New York: Riverhead Books.

Thich Nhat Hanh. 1987. The Miracle of Mindfulness: An Introduction to the Practice of Meditation. Boston: Beacon Press.

Thich Nhat Hanh. 2006. Transformation and Healing: Sutra on the Four Establishments of Mindfulness. Berkeley, California: Parallax Press.

Thich Nhat Hanh. 2001. You Are Here: Discovering the Magic of the Present Moment. Boston & London: Shambhala.

II. The following books specifically address the connections between mindfulness and eating.

Kabatznick, Ronna. 1998. The Zen of Eating: Ancient Answers to Modern Weight Problems. New York: Perigee.

Thich Nhat Hanh & Lilian Cheung. 2010. Savor: Mindful Eating, Mindful Life. New York: HarperOne.

III. I include the following book simply because I think it's the best general self-help book on the market, and a wonderful guide to approaching personal or professional life in a deliberate, mindful way. Over the past twenty years I have re-read this book each time my own life underwent significant change, and have found it wise and helpful each time.

Covey, Stephen R. 1989. <u>The Seven Habits of Highly Effective People: Powerful Lessons in Personal Change</u>. New York: Free Press.

IV. The following book is included as a sample of a genre of "food book" that is becoming more common. It discusses some of the problems associated with "industrial farming," and induces a deeper awareness of our relationship to food in a modern industrial economy.

Pollan, Michael. 2006. <u>The Omnivore's Dilemma: A Natural History of Four Meals.</u> New York: Penguin Books.

Appendix B. RECIPES AND SUGGESTIONS

This appendix is for readers who are not normally cooks or bakers. It's intended to give you suggestions for preparing a few simple items that are easy to fix, healthy, and tasty.

The first is breads.

To start with, here's a basic recipe that I'll expand on afterward.

1 tablespoon active yeast

1 tablespoon sugar or honey

2 cups very warm water

2 cups all-purpose unbleached flour

2 cups whole wheat flour

1 teaspoon salt

Mix the yeast and sugar or honey and the water. Set aside for a few minutes, until it foams up a little. Mix the flours and salt in a separate bowl and then add the liquid mixture. Stir together to make a somewhat thick dough, then dump the dough onto a floured surface and knead it energetically for five minutes or so. Put the dough in an oiled bowl and let it rise in a warm place for an hour. I normally use the oven for this purpose, set to 100 degrees. Then again dump the dough onto a floured surface, break it down into two loaves (or more, if you like small loaves), knead it again, and put it in oiled loaf pans. Let it rise for 20 minutes, then bake for 30 minutes.

The results will be a couple loaves of very simple but surprisingly tasty bread.

But here's the fun part. Using that recipe as the basis, try one or more of the following additions.

1) Add a quarter cup or more of just about any kind of seeds: flaxseed (whole or ground); sesame seeds, sunflower seeds, etc.
2) Add a quarter cup wheat germ.
3) Add half a cup of left over mashed potatoes, cooked oatmeal (preferably steel-cut oats, not rolled oats) or cooked quinoa or couscous.
4) Use the same amount but different kinds of flour. I like to mix oat, barley, soy, rye, spelt, and whatever else catches my eye in the health food store bins.
5) Add half a cup of sautéed onions or leeks or olives (make sure there are no stones).
6) Add one or more of the common flavoring spices: basil, thyme, rosemary, marjoram, sage.
7) Add ¾ cup cranraisins and ¾ cup chopped (not too fine) pecans and a tablespoon or two of cinnamon. This is a spectacular breakfast bread.
8) Dice an apple (Fuji or another firm, flavorful apple), chop ½ cup almonds, add molasses or a mixture of honey and molasses, plus a tablespoon or two of cinnamon, and sautee

over a low heat for ten minutes or so, and add to the basic bread recipe.

These last two variations, when you toast them for breakfast, will make your whole kitchen smell like fresh-baked bread.

You get the idea. Bread is easy and very enjoyable to make and to eat. The variations I have provided are just samples. Bread is very forgiving; you can try almost anything and get a good result.

Second is soups.

I like to make a big pot of soup and have it around for a week of lunches. It's also easy to freeze in meal size portions.

Again I'll start with a very basic soup and then talk about variations.

Rinse a cup of lentils and put them in six to eight cups water or vegetable broth or stock. Add one or two onions and a couple of diced stalks of celery and three or four finely diced garlic cloves. You can add whatever spices you like; I prefer to use a pre-prepared mix of herbs. One I particularly like is Kirkland Brand organic no-salt seasoning, a combination of twenty-one different spices. I think this soup comes out better if you cook it slowly, just hot enough to bubble gently as it cooks. Once the lentils are tender, it's ready. Salt to taste.

That's about as basic a tasty and nourishing soup as you can imagine. I like to puree it in any kind of food processor once it's done.

Here are some ways to jazz it up a little if you prefer.

If you want it a little creamier, add a potato or two.

Add just about any vegetable you want. I use carrots, squash, eggplant, bell peppers, zucchini,and some vegetables I don't recognize from my Thai sister-in-law's back yard garden.

Here's my favorite variation. When the basic recipe, including whatever additional vegetables I have on hand, is ready (i.e., when the lentils and vegetables are tender), add half a cup of uncooked couscous, a cup of tomatoes, and a little less than a tablespoon of curry powder. Cook slowly an additional fifteen minutes, or until the couscous is soft. Puree.

There are many curry powders. Most of them include coriander, turmeric, mustard, chili, ginger, cumin, and fenugreek, and some add other herbs. Of the ones I've tried, my favorite is called "Indo-European Madras Curry Powder." It comes in a pint jar, and is made by Indo-European Foods, Inc. of Glendale, California.

Finally, breakfast.

Did you know that breakfast can be the most important meal of the day in terms of diet and health?

When my wife and I get up in the morning, our first order of business is to decide what we want for breakfast. It's usually one of four: omelets; steel-cut oats with raisins or frozen mixed berries and honey; pecan/blueberry pancakes; or French toast with sliced sautéed pear with maple syrup. The first two I usually make; the second two she normally does.

By far the most frequent consensus is omelets. That sounds plain and simple, but let me tell you about the variations. The base of all our omelets is just one egg, a little almond milk, and salt and pepper.

We've both gotten very fond of spinach omelets, but for my wife's, I start by sautéing a slice of red onion, diced, until it's tender, then I add spinach leaves with the stems trimmed off and sautee the onion and spinach together for a minute or so. Then I add the egg, almond milk, salt and pepper, along with a couple slices of avocado, diced, and one piece of defatted bacon, diced. This omelet, along with a couple slices of my cranraisin pecan cinnamon toast, guarantees a happy customer. Since my wife is allergic to dairy products the avocado is an excellent substitute for cheese.

But again, there are plenty of other variations you can substitute. One I like is the basic ingredients, plus spinach, plus a diced slice of tomato, cheddar cheese, and either a diced slice of ham or one diced link sausage.

My main message underlying this food appendix is that mindfulness about food can extend to its preparation. Some people I've talked to about weight management equate managing weight with bland, unsatisfying diets. They think of losing weight as a painful or at least unpleasant drill that takes all the pleasure out of eating. Mindful management of our diet can be just the opposite. It can focus everything we know or learn about our bodies and their nourishment in a way that adds to our whole experience of food preparation and consumption.

www.ingramcontent.com/pod-product-compliance
Lightning Source LLC
Chambersburg PA
CBHW060522290526
45791CB00001B/493